Preface

Congratulations, yes, you heard it right. It's me, the book in your hand, talking to you.

Please listen carefully. Many people may find what I am about to tell them strange, unfamiliar, and even counterintuitive. Despite this, I will still disclose this secret that has been kept from you. This will eventually reach your heart, and it will reveal that you are born brilliant and intelligent. You have the potential to reach remarkable heights. All that is needed is to unlock the power of the mind within. The way you can do it and will do it is what I'm going to tell you because I have been written after years of research about how a brain can produce the best interface of intelligence and creativity.

There is a secret that you should know your intelligence and incredible creative abilities are hidden in several regions of your brain. The wonders inside are screaming to you through the rusted doors of your mind, but you are programmed in such a way that you cannot hear them.

Since my author is a neurologist, he has studied not only the intellectual abilities of geniuses, scientists, philosophers, and thinkers throughout history. he has also dug into their secrets by studying what makes their brain function at its peak. He has discovered how these remarkable people's creative process differs from the average person's. Additionally, he has discovered how to enhance your brain's efficiency by applying the same simple techniques that these geniuses employed. In this way, you will be able to access a reservoir of knowledge and ideas that you would not otherwise be able to access

Dedicated to my mother,
a person who has always
been there for me.

I am grateful for her
love. She is the reason I
have become the person
I am today.

INDEX

Step 1	
Let's find out The optimal state of your super- energised mind. Research-based revelations	38
Chapter content	
Can we increase the mind's thinking and intelligence capabilities by 500%? What is the most powerful mind state? What are the steps to achieving this? What can this research of mine do for you? My study of the lives of the world's significant achievers and icons of self-actualisation has led me to which conclusion? Are you aware that you are innately intelligent? Imagine how much faster you could develop mind skills if you knew how to use revolutionary research to accelerate your progress. The mystery of history's greatest creators and geniuses is revealed.	39 - 53

Step 2	
Explore the mysterious secrets of history's master artists, scientists, and geniuses. Apply it easily to your mind	54
Chapter content	
What made Shakespeare, Rumi and Iqbal able to write millions of poetic pieces in such a short period of time? This secret needs to be revealed. Is it possible to bring ideas to the shore of your mind like the waves of the sea? How can we do that? In my experience as a neurologist, I can tell you who can achieve the superstate! Can anyone at any age achieve it? This book will reveal the secret behind what was once thought to be a mysterious skill of artists, poets, scientists, and geniuses. What the flow state can reveal about your mind's brilliance? How can a flow state make you successful in your role in life? Is there a reason why Einstein did not use the prevailing thinking methods? In what way can you induce such a thinking process in yourself? Find new ways to succeed by visualising ideas rather than using words.	55 - 66

Step 3	
Discover the state of mind of the world's most successful individuals	67
Chapter content	
Is there anything sadder than seeing people perform below their potential? What causes so many people to fail? Is there a common cause? Can a flow state provide a glimpse of the future? Is there anything we can learn from the marshmallow test? Is there anything it reveals? What is the connection between flow and success, and how does it facilitate it?	68 - 76

Step 4	
Here is a message from the Free Climbers sharing their successful strategies. A look at who they are and what we can learn from them?	77
Chapter content	
Those who climb mountains on their own without any assistance. They send a message that you should pay attention to If you take every step of life as if it guarantees your survival, you will give the utmost importance to every step of your life. What is the best way to reach the top of your life? How can deep focus be achieved?	78 - 83

Step 5	
Identifying the most successful players' minds	84
Chapter content	
How can a flow state break through comfort zone barriers? How did this man climb Mount Everest wearing shorts in extreme cold? You also have that power. Let us learn about Usain Bolt's journey to becoming one of the best athletes in the world. He achieved this feat by relentlessly pushing his flow state to new limits. How to overcome the fear of winning and losing? How best athletes and players do this to achieve the best performance by doing that. What we can learn? What do great players like Bradman and Tiger Wood have in common?	85 - 95

Step 6	
Is there a brain king who rules us? Discovering the hidden intelligence that has been suppressed and how to regain it	96
Chapter content	
What is the part of our brain that governs the mind? And keeps us in a logical box. How is freedom from this possible? One more secret you should know: intelligence exists in many other areas and places in the brain. Due to the dictator of this brain, many intelligent areas of our mind are under control. How to free these intelligent areas of our brain? How the great genius scientist, poets, and thinkers defeats this dictator of his mind After flow waves silence the prefrontal cortex's rule, the suppressed intelligence areas are now independent	97 - 106

Step 7	
Your brain works like a radio, learn and hack it	107
Chapter content	
It may surprise you that the brain is also an electrical machine. It uses electrical signals to communicate with the rest of the body. These signals allow us to think, move, feel, and remember.

How can high-quality electrical currents and electrical waves work best? To ensure proper electrical currents, what do we need to do?

How do brain surface waves affect the brain in terms of its function?

The way the brain selects its channels is like how a radio selects its channels.

Brain surface waves are rhythmic patterns of electrical activity produced by neurons in the brain. These waves help the brain to select the most relevant signals. How to get the best wave and best current? | 108 - 115 |

# Step 9	
Here are your most powerful brain chemicals. Find out which cocktail is the best and how to get it?	127
## Chapter content	
During flow states, which neurochemicals serve as cement for rebuilding your brain?	128 - 137
You can create and use superfast mind tracks when these brain-produced chemicals are released during flow.	
Dopamine causes your success, and it is the one brain chemical which can cause your failure.	
Let me introduce you to a very interesting. chemicals that you have in your brain. Anandamide. The word is derived from the Sanskrit term "Ananda", which means "bliss".	
Engaging in a flow state increases Dopamine naturally and promotes the release of the finest blend of chemicals	
This also answers an intriguing question I have had in my mind for years. Now I know why a painter, a poet or a philosopher becomes addicted to their work	

Step 11	
The best way to come up with ideas without overthinking	146
Chapter content	
Ideas are like dreams. How do they come about? Your thinking perception will never be the same after you hear my hypothesis. It is estimated that there are seventy thousand thoughts in a day, but what if there was even one idea? The best ideas can come to you like dreams during waking hours. Learn the technique. When you sleep, do you construct your dreams? What will we learn from the answer to this question? How is it possible to generate ideas, the highest thoughts, in one's mind without overthinking them? Suppose a situation in which, in front of your eyes, a building and its walls were created automatically without a single worker being present. Can the buildings of creation in your mind be built like that? Great ideas and general thoughts - what is the difference? Nothing can stop you from succeeding if you know this.	147 - 155

Step 13	
Identifying the single most important factor for success. Let's figure out the easiest way to focus	164
Chapter content	
What is the importance of focusing on focus? Make your success possible with research? Why is it important to pay attention to yourself? Why is your focus the most responsible for your success? A big revelation. Bird's Eye is a story of thousands of years and its hidden secret. How can you befriend your rights and make them your slaves? Who will do for you what no one else can?	165 - 173

Step 14	
Explore the relationship between your thoughts and your focus of mind. What you can do to take control?	174
## Chapter content	
You're about to discover an exciting way to connect your thoughts, mind, and focus. There are endless possibilities. How do you expand the horizons of your mind? An idea or sensation stretches a man's mind and never sprints back to its former dimensions. Are you looking to broaden your perspective and strengthen your relationship with yourself? All of us have a major sense of disbelief about ourselves.	175 - 182

Step 15	
Why do we experience intense power in the flow state? How does it allow us to reach peak performance?	183
Chapter content	
Nature's golden law and secret: energy flows in directions where there is flow. What can you do to enhance your intelligence by using this law? What is the importance of mental flow? The rapture of our minds and hearts is like a leaf on the waves of a river. Why do we need it? Is it possible to create the most powerful waves of our mind just as easily as they are in the ocean? A small fish in the Atlantic Ocean can withstand waves nine feet high with the power it generates. How can we provide that kind of power?	184 - 193

Step 16	
Walk like Darwin to think Like Darwin How walks get you in Zone and can make you super intelligent	194
Chapter content	
There comes a point when you start reading your hidden mind while you are walking; why do you reach that point in your walking? The switch of ideas is turned on by walking. But how? A look at how walking transformed Charles Dickens and William Wordsworth and other geniuses. During walking, what precious neurochemicals and growth factors are released? Research reveals how walking affects the size of people's brains even over age 60.	195 - 205

Step 17	
A hidden power of Mother Earth's electromagnetic energy that can influence our minds must be revealed	206
Chapter content	
No one has ever told you about the power of the Earth that you can use for your mind and thinking. Your current location influences how you think. How does it affect your thinking and mind? Electrical energy can be found on Earth's surface in what ways? Introducing Showman Resonance, an amazing scientific secret. In what ways can electromagnetic waves around the Earth affect our brains? Amasing research? Get in touch with Mother Earth again, but why?	207 - 216

Step 18	
Getting the best out of our brain during the Divine Hours of the Night- How it works?	217
Chapter content	
Do the hours between three and five in the night have any power? Could it be due to the electromagnetic field network? During this period, you can experience a heightened awareness of the energy around you.	218 - 228
Which makes this time of night powerful? This time is known as the 'Divine Hour'. It is the time when the veil between the physical and spiritual worlds is thinnest.	
How did my father, Sehba Akhtar, use this hour of the night for rapture poetry? He would sit atop a creative hill and write, letting the Divine Hour energy flow through him and onto the paper.	
What is the point of spending one night a week alone with a pen and paper? In a special way, the quietness of the night, coupled with the creative energy of the hour, will allow you to tap into his innermost thoughts and feelings.	

Step 19	
Getting great ideas, one of the best times of the day What is happening in our brain just before we completely wake up?	229
Chapter content	
Since birth till now the most precious time of your day is easily wasted by you. Why did Edison and Tesla etc. sleep holding an iron ball before going to sleep? "And why is there ever a need to leave the feeling of now? How should one use the powerful waves of the mind immediately after waking up?	230 - 238

Step 20	
Thinking with closed eyes: why does it work for geniuses and how will it work for you?	239
Chapter content	
Have you seen the pictures of Einstein and Alama Iqbal thinking while closed-eyed? Do geniuses and thinkers often think with their eyes closed? When recalling a memory, why do people close their eyes? The secret reveals what happens to our brain waves when we close our eyes and think!	240 - 249

Step 21	
Discover the wonders of daydreaming - Visualise your daydreams every day, but why?	250
Chapter content	
Despite being wide awake, you start dreaming, but why? Based on my research on daydreaming, here's a tip for you. Daydreaming can assist your brain in processing creative solutions to challenges. A novel concept I have developed is called "Day dream meditation." Dream meditation is consciously directing one's thoughts and imagination to access creative ideas and solutions—a powerful tool for tapping into the subconscious mind and uncovering hidden potential. How did Einstein's daydreams change our world forever? He famously visualised himself riding on a beam of light, which led him to develop special relativity theory. Are you interested in finding out how to access the most intelligent parts of your brain? Are you curious about unlocking your hidden potential? Try closing your eyes and dreaming of success, but why? We can use them to push us to strive for our goals and take the first steps toward achieving our ambitions.	251 - 261

Step 22	
An innovative hypothesis for driving intelligence: connecting to the past, present, and future creative auras	262
Chapter content	
What is an aura or halo of power around us? And how is it created? How can the aura of energy around highly intelligent people and those who are at the pinnacle of their craft empower your mind? How can it benefit you to be in the company or company of such people? Can these geniuses and masters of their art send waves of wisdom to your brain on how this theory of mine can surprisingly benefit you? When thousands of millions of birds flying in the sky, without talking to each other, how do they go around in a circle with great speed? Amasing revelation.	263 - 273

Step 23	
Master the mind's mastering flow by unraveling mystical mental codes	274
Chapter content	
Where is the key to your mental treasures? How can words and phrases magically become keys to the treasures of the mind? If we have to open the closed doors of the mind and their locks, what flames must be awakened in our mind? And how will they melt the chains binding the mind, but how? Based on the research you will find.	275 - 280

Step 24	
A way to disconnect for ultimate connection with Darvish Sufi Dance - Elevate your mind with this new paradigm	281
Chapter content	
Let's find out about a state of mind far more powerful than sleeping and waking. What was the reason for Maulana Rum's invention of Sufi dance? Does it have any mind-boosting properties? How can one spin in a circle 24 times a minute during the Sufi Dance of Dervishes? Like a planet, the flowing movements connect to the ultimate forces of the universe. Is there a scientific explanation for how Buddha reached Nirvana? let's find out. How was this state of awareness made possible by the flow of the mind? What is the reason that spiritual experiences and situations cannot be described in words? What brainwave can take you to your deepest layers?	282 - 292

Step 25	
Think Like a Child and act like an adult - unlock your own creativity	293
Chapter content	
As we grow older, do we lose the sense of wonder and curiosity we once had as children? Do we know why? Could we be able to reclaim the power of imagination we had as children as we age? To realise our potential, does it make sense to see the world through the eyes of a child? Does there exist a reason why children do not have a time-scarcity mindset? In what ways can we apply the golden rule through the flow state? What can children teach us about getting into a Flow State distinctively and seamlessly?	294 - 303

# Step 27	
How to utlise impact of your room on your thinking, Creating a creative and productive environment?	317
## Chapter content	
In your life, where do you spend the most of your time? There is so much more to your room than just walls and ceilings that you should make it yours. Your room's walls and doors can transmit the most powerful messages to you What is the importance of the room being bright, colourful, smelling good, hearing good, and having a good view? Your living room needs a living, breathing plant. There should always be three books next to your bed in your room.	318 - 326

Step 28	
The magical effects of music on the brain - How to use music to boost your brain waves	327
Chapter content	
Is it true that everything in the universe is always in flux? What can we gain by knowing that every particle of our body has a flow within it? How much power is there in music and tones? Through his music and raga, Tansen made it rain and lit up the extinguished lamps, but how? What are the findings of a study on the brains of 9,000 musicians? What is the mechanism by which the sound of music activates the powerful waves of our mind?	328 - 337

Step 29	
How Shower can instigate brilliant ideas — learn the trick	338
Chapter content	
You probably don't know that you have slow, fast, and super-fast tracks of thinking. Do you? How can the slow, fast, and super-fast brain pathways of thinking can be used? What other surprising changes does taking a shower make to the surface of our brains that we can use for our ideas? What was the Archimedes Eureka moment? And how can we create eureka moments in our lives? How can Aqua Notes be used while bathing? How and why does a new idea suddenly jump to the surface of the mind while taking a shower? How can we use it in our practical life?	339 - 349

Step 30	
How to use super power of collective consciousness?	350
Chapter content	
What is "C" energy that can be found in libraries or other places where people engage in collective thinking? What is a 3C phenomenon, according to me? By understanding this, you can create an optimal electromagnetic environment for your brain. How does our brain's default setting work? How do focused people create an energised environment around them?	251 - 257

Step 31	
Four superpower stages to your mystical flow	358
Chapter content	
What four important steps are necessary to bring us into mental flow? In order to get into mental flow, one must first set a goal. And then forget this goal and immerse yourself in the steps and steps taken for it, but how? You must use your mind in a certain way. Let's find out next. How not to build dams in front of flowing ideas. How to stop the newscaster of your mind? Why is it important to keep the flame of emotions low in mental flow?	259 - 368

Step 32	
Supercharge your brain by learning breathing patterns?	369
Chapter content	
How can the brain be supercharged in five seconds? Let's learn together. A new way of breathing is possible. What are the ways in which breathing can change the way we think and feel? What are the two wires (nerves) in your chest that control? your breathing and thinking? Let's know the secret. How a unique Breathing method Can Superfast Your Brain Let's explore this research.	370 - 377

You have wasted your most precious time of the day since you were born, so it's no wonder why you are so easily distracted.

The iron ball was held by Edison and other geniuses before they went to sleep. Why did they do this?

How should one use the powerful waves of the mind immediately after waking up?

Step 1

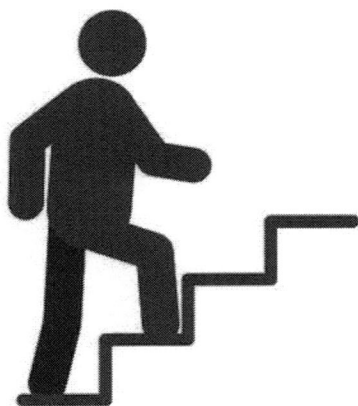

Let's find out The optimal state of your super-energised mind. Research-based revelations

In next few pages
you're about to find out!

- Can we increase the mind's thinking and intelligence capabilities by 500%?

- What is the most powerful mind state? What are the steps to achieving this? What can this research of mine do for you?

- My study of the lives of the world's significant achievers and icons of self-actualisation has led me to which conclusion?

- Are you aware that you are innately intelligent? Imagine how much faster you could develop mind skills if you knew how to

use revolutionary research to
accelerate your progress.

- The mystery of history's greatest
  creators and geniuses is revealed.

After researching the scientific literature and the lives of great thinkers, brilliant artists, and extraordinary scientists over the years, I have concluded that one common factor they have all used is to increase the power of the mind by up to five hundred per cent. This is a super powerful state of mind, the "Magical flow state of mind."

This state of mind can allow individuals to access their full creative potential and is a key factor in achieving success in any field.

As a Neurologist, I can tell you that anyone can achieve this superstate at any age, regardless of IQ level. Our magical mind is just a few steps away, so let's start. I can confirm It is not difficult at all. All it takes is dedication and the proper techniques, and you can begin harnessing the power of your mind to reach this superstate.

This superstate is achievable by anyone and everyone and can provide amazing results. All that is required is knowledge of the techniques and the commitment to practising them on a daily basis. With practice, you can become the master of your own mind and achieve success.

Think carefully about the way you spend your time. On average, how many hours of work do you do each day? As a result of neuroscience research, we can demonstrate that you can permanently change your life after attaining this super state of mind. Imagine learning

After researching the scientific Literature and the Lives of great thinkers, brilliant artists and extraordinary scientists over the years, I have concluded that one common factor they have all used is to increase the power of the mind by up to five hundred per cent.

anything at a rate of five hundred per cent, regardless of what you wish to learn.

Now we know the secret behind what once was considered a mysterious skill of artists, philosophers, painters, and other geniuses. We can now use this newfound knowledge to unlock our creative potential and express ourselves in ways we never thought possible. Having knowledge of these secrets will not only allow us to explore and discover new aspects of our own minds but also help us shape our future outlook.

Now we know the **secret** behind **what** once **was considered** a mysterious **skill** of **artists,** philosophers, painters, **and** other **geniuses.**

Based on Neuroscientific evidence, almost everyone can develop such deep creativity and productivity. It would help if you learned the art of achieving a flow state to create new and better ideas. Like the heads of a melody and the sequence and flow of counting numbers, the strings of ideas in the flow state are intertwined.

One idea follows another, followed by another, then by a third, then a fourth, then a fifth, and finally by five hundred and one. The flow of ideas remains constant and seamless without much hindrance. An uninterrupted stream of ideas yields a continuous pattern, interlinking and evolving in an ever-evolving manner that never ceases to amaze.

The same subject unifies thoughts and their flow. There is no interruption. If you are in a flow state while performing any task, physical or mental, you will become so engrossed that you will not be distracted by anything else. Neither the external nor the internal, not even you, could stand in the way of your harmonious flow of ideas and activities when you are in it.

As a result of this state of magical mind spellbinding, you will be at the top of your game and will be a peak performer in your life. This state of mind is a powerful tool that can be used to become a master of any craft; it's the key to achieving success and reaching your fullest potential.

The flow state is characterised by electrochemical changes that produce super electrical waves in the brain. This type of electromagnetic activity helps to create intense creativity, and clarity - a state often associated with peak performance. These electrical waves, in turn, result in a state of heightened focus and awareness that is often referred to as being "in the zone".

> **Once you** reach a **flow state, you can discover your mind's hidden brilliance.** You **will be in** your **most productive self in the flow**

This state of peak performance can help you accomplish tasks more efficiently, allowing you to reach success more quickly. After one achieves a flow state, any physical or mental task becomes so engaging that no one is bothered by anything like, time, place, or even oneself. Are you aware of what you don't know about yourself? You can find hidden thoughts in your mind. You can also discover your hidden talents.

Once you reach a flow state, you can discover your mind's hidden brilliance. You will be in your most productive self in the flow state. And once you have forgotten everything, you will be so absorbed with this work that the string of the previous thought binds your every review. The continuity of the subject and focus will remain intact. Everything that occurs is inextricably linked to everything that follows.

My experience as a Neurologist tells me that when you attain this state, the most powerful waves in your brain begin to move. A flow state is an experience in which no hard work is felt after completing a task. It becomes effortless. Your work becomes seamless. Your pen glides effortlessly across the page. The ideas just flowed to you. You didn't have. to look hard to find them. Nor you took a hammer and a chisel and use them on any stone. But the shape of the statue itself came to the fore.

"

What is the most
powerful mind state?
What are the steps
to achieving this?

What can this
research of mine do
for you?

"

DNA

You will become ......

You will
become so
engrossed that you
will not be
distracted by
anything else.
Neither the
external nor the
internal,
not even you, could
stand in the way of
your harmonious
flow
of ideas

DNA

In sports, extensive records couldn't be broken because people couldn't give their best because of their mental prison.

The individuals who could break the chains of thinking became engrossed in a flow state and made many records. One psychologist identified the state of mind known as the superpower flow for the first time in 1975. In his opinion, the person who performs the work in the flow state is completely immersed in the work process with total concentration and wholly absorbed in it.

As a result, the person is cut off from where they are and from time. With the revolutionary information we receive from our neuroscience experiments, we have access to the answers that were not available to us fifteen years ago. In other words, if we don't use this information, then we're being ungrateful for God's blessings.

Most Likely, you are unaware that your mind **contains several great ideas.** When you **experience** this unique state of mind, you can **uncover all the secret thoughts** in your mind.

Most likely, you are unaware that your mind contains several great ideas. When you experience this unique state of mind, you can uncover all the secret thoughts in your mind. By doing so, you will discover your hidden talents. Your mental strength is something you do not know about! No matter what subject you are working on, whether you're trying to solve an algebraic equation or a painting technique.

Whether you are sitting in an exam room, solving papers, or running 100 meters on the track. No matter what you do, your performance will increase by 200 to 500 percent. Your mind will reveal its hidden

You can do whatever you want after it has been incorporated into your mind.
You are free to Learn

brilliance once it reaches a flow state. Your mind will be at its most potent and productive mode. The other essential thing is that you have lived with extraordinary mental energy and abilities since birth.

However, they have yet to be utilised. This book aims to help us understand the flow state and its potential so that we can use it in our lives. There's no need to worry. It's super simple. It may be challenging at first since it takes time to get started. Once you begin the process, you'll see the possibilities. You'll get in the habit of using flow state mode.

If you reach this state, you can access the hidden powers within you or those hidden in your subconscious. Why does your intelligence increase while in the flow state? For example, the intelligence centres of your brain that you have not previously utilised will begin to activate. Your subconscious mind can start using these intelligence centres, which you have never used.

You can focus with extreme speed, a speed you didn't anticipate. You can design and build bullet trains of your ideas using the tracks in your brain. An entirely new circuit of intelligence will be constructed. Intelligence tracks and circuits will start forming and activating areas of your brain that you hadn't previously activated. One

You can focus ......

You can
focus with
extreme speed, a
speed you didn't
anticipate. You
can design and
build bullet
train of your
ideas using the
tracks in your
brain.
An entirely new
circuit of
intelligence will
be constructed.

DNA

example is activating the parts of your brain that you have not used before, such as your intelligence centres. Your subconscious mind will increase your thinking speed by five hundred percent by using something you have never used before.

There is another angle to why flow state is best: divine flow permeates everything. We will realize that everything around us is flowing if we take the time to reflect. Rivers, seas, and air all are in the flow. The clouds float in the sky. As we stand on the earth now, it is in a state of flow and spinning. Planets orbit the sun and are in flow, and when we look inside, we see that our breathing is also a form of flow. Blood circulates in our bodies in a flow.

A quantum particle of an object is directly in front of us, yet invisible to the naked eye, is in the flow. Atoms' electrons are constantly in flux. There is nothing more divine than flow. Everything in our existence is in flow.

It is the society that convinces us of our reality. But is society always right? The world expects us to be averagely intelligent and incapable of imagining big things. There must be an end to this fearful idea, which is artificial and completely erroneous.

> A quantum particle of an object is directly in front of us, yet invisible to the naked eye, is in the flow. Atoms' electrons are constantly in flux. There is nothing more divine than flow.

You can break this chain of these hindrances. I assure you, you can. All you have to do is to decide. Society's opinions about you or how they make you feel aren't always the right thing to listen to. You may need to be made aware of this fact. When you look in the mirror in the morning, what you see is your reflection. This mirror's reflection does not reveal the successful person hidden inside you. This person will eventually be revealed to you. Ultimately, you will discover it for yourself. A flow state could be a means of presenting it to the world.

> A person can achieve this mental flow at any age or intelligence level. Everyone can gain it gradually

The book will help dispel misconceptions that people cannot be intelligent or can't think big. It is an entirely false and artificial fear, and its chain must be broken. And believe me, it can be broken. You can break the chains if you decide to. Society does not always know what it tells you about yourself or makes you feel.

If you dare to think outside the box, this book will surely help you find yourself. Looking in the mirror in the morning, you only see yourself reflected. You have not been looking for the successful person hidden inside you in the reflection of this mirror. Nevertheless, this successful person can be found if you search for him. And you can make it happen for yourself. You can also present it to the world through a flow state.

It's fascinating to realise that you have already experienced this flow state without ever knowing it. It may surprise you, but let me remind you. Think back to when you were young and involved in sports. Your full attention, focus, and the whole waves of your brain are devoted to the game and its decisions. The same goes for watching an exciting movie. Whether watching a film, reading a book, or listening to your favourite music, until the credits roll, you will not even realise how much time has passed. Flow states allow you to become completely immersed in whatever you are doing. During this time, during this activity, your brain forms mighty waves.

Generally, such powerful waves are only used during leisure or entertainment activities. Electrical waves can be used to generate great ideas and in the production of great thought. This can help our brains become more creative. Using these waves to guide our learning will help us go a long way. Success lies in the flow of deep focus. This is why mastering this skill is vital for success.

The book will help dispel misconceptions that people cannot be or can't think big. It is an entirely

Success Lies in......

Success Lies in the
flow of deep focus.
This is why
mastering this skill
is vital for success.
Our research found
that focus is like a
laser beam that gets
brighter and dimmer
with time.

DNA

Step 2

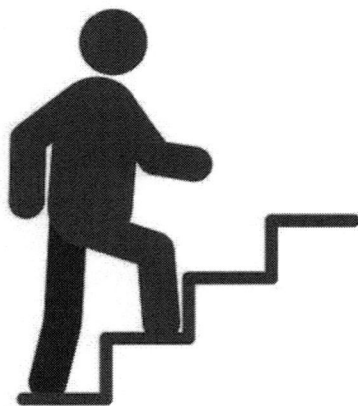

Explore the mysterious secrets of history's master artists, scientists, and geniuses, Apply it easily to your mind

In next few pages
you're about to find out!

- What made Shakespeare, Rumi and Iqbal able to write millions of poetic pieces in such a short period of time? This secret needs to be revealed.

- Is it possible to bring ideas to the shore of your mind like the waves of the sea? How can we do that?

- In my experience as a neurologist, I can tell you who can achieve the superstate! Can anyone at any age achieve it?

- This book will reveal the secret behind what was once thought to be a mysterious skill of artists, poets, scientists, and geniuses.

- What the flow state can reveal about your mind's brilliance?

- How can a flow state make you successful in your role in life?

- Is there a reason why Einstein did not use the prevailing thinking methods? In what way can you induce such a thinking process in yourself?

- Find new ways to succeed by visualising ideas rather than using words.

Throughout history, brilliant artists and scientists have used flow states to create their art and discoveries. Irrespective of whether he is a celebrated poet like Ghalib or a prominent sufi like Rumi. Works of art, inventions, or poetry. People who write verses, write ghazals, or those who paint, or those who play sports. In order to perform at their highest level, they must land in a certain zone.

Certainly, all these geniuses use flow state to maximise their productivity, i.e., to accomplish their creations. Throughout history, we find many examples of what happens to people when they enter the flow state.

During the writing of Principia Mathematica, Newton says he forgot to eat, drink, or bathe. When Michelangelo painted, he attained a state of flow, which he would refer to as painting in a flow state. So, he would also be in a flow like Newton.

Look at the state of mind of all these magnificent creators of history for a moment, and you will see what I mean. As a result, you can see how much of a creative contribution they have made in their short lives.

Here, I want you to know an invaluable secret. Scientists have found that some brain waves can create novel thoughts and ideas in the mind of an individual that are not possible in a normal state of mind. They are in alpha and theta states, respectively.

> During the writing of Principia Mathematica, Newton says he forgot to eat, drink, or bathe. When Michelangelo painted, he attained a state of flow which he would refer to as painting in a flow state. So he would also be in a flow like Newton.

Neuroscience tells us that certain brain waves are so powerful that they facilitate the creation of novel and unique thoughts and ideas, thoughts and ideas that cannot be achieved in a normal state of mind. These brain waves are called alpha waves and theta waves. The purpose of this book will be to explain in greater detail how you can achieve this state of mind through various exercises.

> There will be rare and **unique ideas** that will occur **spontaneously. During the process** of Alpha and theta state of mind, creative ideas and **unique** perspectives emerge as if **ripples** in a river.

Learning these exercises is not difficult. It is possible to transform our ordinary lives into extraordinary ones if we know these secrets. We will delve into these exercises in much more detail later in the book.

Take a look at the Masnavi of Maulana Rumi and see how many poems are in it. Upon reading Iqbal's poems, you will notice that they are not the work of an ordinary person. In terms of science, let me state that this is not a matter of an ordinary or exceptional individual. It is a way of thinking that enables any individual to prepare his or her mind in such a manner that he or she can automatically grasp rare and excellent ideas in a relaxed and automatic state of mind. There will be rare and unique ideas that will occur spontaneously. During the process of Alpha and theta state of mind, creative ideas and unique perspectives emerge as if ripples in a river.

Let me give you other examples from history to convince you. Through conventional thinking, Einstein could never have discovered what he discovered in his lifetime. Einstein sought out discoveries and creative ideas while using the flow state of mind instead of thinking like 99.9% of the world's population. The early years of Einstein's life were remarkable and beyond comprehension.

Besides conceptualizing ideas verbally, he also visualized them.

"

Is it possible to
bring ideas to the
shore of your mind
like the waves of
the sea? How can we
do that?

"

DNA

There was a very popular experiment in which celestial lightning collided with a moving train, and free-fall experiments from a dynamic descending elevator became very popular. Geniuses often use a method called visual thinking.

Einstein was working on his theory of relativity in 1915. Albert Einstein was disturbed to learn that one of his students was about to surpass him in terms of research. In lieu of ignoring this difficulty, he chose to focus on what he was an expert in. In order to solve each of the challenges, he divided them into stages and concentrated on one aspect of the task at hand. He would not change his mind unless he were not successful.

> **Einstein was working on his theory of relativity in 1915.** Albert Einstein was **disturbed to learn that one of his** students was **about to surpass him in terms of** research

He was deeply engrossed in the project and eager to complete it. Then, he imposed a condition on himself in which he would utilise the most powerful electric waves of his brain. He would enter a trance in which he could solve his equations. Spending hours at his study table isolated from people, he would concentrate his thinking at one point and find the answer to his questions. For hours, he would devote himself to the answers to his questions.

Every morning, Einstein was always in a superpower state of mind. During his morning walks in the park, he would supercharge his brain.

We should recognise that our attention and focus are no different from those of a wild horse. A wild horse cannot be tamed overnight. Taming horses require time and effort. Gradually, though, the wild horse of your attention can be trained using different techniques. Then we can embark on a journey of success on this fast horse of

"

This book will reveal the secret behind what was once thought to be a mysterious skill of artists, poets, scientists and geniuses.

"

DNA

ours. A flow state is an excellent way to control your attention.

This book aims to provide as much information as possible about the most powerful electric waves of the mind. This will allow us to unlock the secrets of supreme intelligence. Electric waves can be transmitted to the surface of the brain. It is not difficult to activate different parts of the brain that have intelligence.

Several centuries ago, a human being could not be contained within a single field. An individual could be both an artist and a scientist. There is a general belief today that artists and scientists are at odds with each other. At Da Vinci, both aspects merged to such an extent that it was difficult to distinguish between him as a scientist and an artist.

Among his artworks, around fifteen are still in existence. In particular, his paintings of the Mona Lisa and The Last Supper are considered immortal despite his significant contributions to botany, architecture, engineering, engraving, geology, astronomy, music, philosophy, and mathematics. Leonardo Da Vinci's Mona Lisa painting is the most famous. For centuries, people have been fascinated by this painting, which was completed in 1516. The mysterious smile of the woman in the painting intrigues them.

My assessment indicates that the individual was highly energetic and used the flow state efficiently. He would use his left hand whenever he desired and his right hand whenever he desired. In order to maintain the secrecy of some of his scripts, he would write from his right side. The scripts could only be read in a mirror's reflection. Thus, they are referred to as mirror writings. At the same time, he could write with both his left and right hands simultaneously.

As a neurologist, I can tell you

That this activity can stimulate both major areas of the brain, thus, the most powerful electric waves can be transmitted to the surface of the brain.

It is not difficult to activate different parts of the brain that have intelligence.

DNA

Think of how many brain neurons a person must use to put them into action and accomplish extraordinary things. The flow state of mind is definitely evident in this process.

In Leonardo's study, there is a great deal of depth. Leonardo took the time to look deeply into his surroundings. Historiographer Vasari once wrote that if he saw something interesting in someone's face, he would follow that person for the whole day and observe it from all angles. Vasari's work alone encompasses 13,000 pages because he observed daily life from all angles.

This, too, reflects a state of flow. Approximately 2 to 3 percent of a person's mental capacity is used on average. A prisoner-like shell surrounds him. Eventually, it reaches the end. Imagine how the world would change if the normal brain, which has been locked inside its shell, was allowed to operate at 100% capacity. Undoubtedly, life and man will reach the point of development where ecstasy is possible.

Please note that even if you are not an artist, a poet, a philosopher, or a scientist, you are still a student of life. Let's assume you are not interested in becoming Leonardo Da Vinci, Michelangelo, Ghalib, Rumi, or Einstein. You are, however, becoming something. You have some connection to the world of work. There is something you are doing in your daily life. Then you should definitely enter the flow state of mind. We need to uncover a few secrets to understand the brain's secret mode and state of flow. These secrets are not as difficult as they appear. Unfortunately, no one has told you about them.

No attempt has ever been undertaken to unravel these secrets. Specifically, how is it possible for a man to possess intelligence? For instance, what makes a person like us more creative? What makes him Leonardo Da Vinci? What caused him to become Michelangelo? In what way did he become Rumi, Ghalib, or Einstein? Formerly, we believed geniuses were born. They cannot be created. Not anymore. Everyone told us this, so we believed them. In the same way that leaders are born and not created, we are also told that some gifted people can accomplish some remarkable things. Therefore, we bowed our heads before them.

We have made no attempt to unravel these secrets.

Specifically, how is it possible for a man to possess intelligence? For instance, what makes a person like us more creative?

What makes him Leonardo Da Vinci? What caused him to become Michelangelo? In what way did he become Rumi, Ghalib, or Einstein?

DNA

Step 3

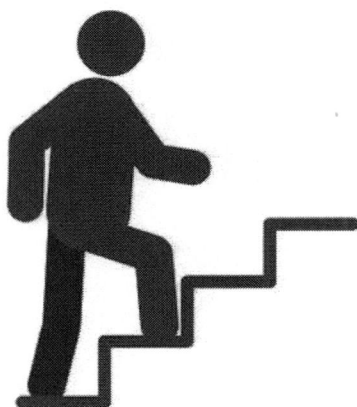

Discover the state of mind of the world's most successful individuals

In next few pages
you're about to find out!

- Is there anything sadder than seeing people perform below their potential?

- What causes so many people to fail? Is there a common cause?

- Can a flow state provide a glimpse of the future?

- Is there anything we can learn from the marshmallow test? Is there anything it reveals?

- What is the connection between flow and success, and how does it facilitate it?

Nothing saddens me more than seeing people living their lives below their true potential. It is as if they are trapped in an uninspiring and unfulfilling existence. As a result of years spent researching the human mind's potential, I have learned how imperative it is to make tough decisions by using the flow of the mind. Furthermore, I've learned that success requires letting go of unproductive and indecisive states. The flow state helps you generate decisions which you were finding difficult to reach.

Flow state does not allow your turtle brain to control your thoughts and actions - rather, it helps you to take charge and start acting on instincts as all successful people in the world do.

Many people fail because they are afraid to fail; when they are afraid of failing, they don't start things in the first place. It is my belief that the one way to be successful is by making mistakes, which is why we are firm believers in the philosophy WTF (Willing to Fail). Flow takes the fear of failure away.

The flow state assists successful individuals in creating a clear vision of their future and providing direction. Without a clear and compelling vision for your long-term goals, you will not be motivated to stay on track over a lengthy period.

In spite of the fact that successful people come from all walks of life, they all share one thing in common: they see challenges as

Nothing saddens me more than seeing people living their lives below their true potential. It is as if they are trapped in an uninspiring and unfulfilling existence.

Many people fail because ......

Many people fail
because they are
afraid to fail,
and when they
are afraid of
failing, they
don't start
things in the
first place - It is
my belief that the
one way to be
successful is by
making mistakes
but not repeating them.

DNA

"

What causes so many
people to fail? Is
there a common
cause?
"

DNA

opportunities to embrace and obstacles to overcome. It's no secret that many successful people share similar thought patterns. Expecting to be able to succeed without a plan or strategy is equivalent to embarking on survival camping on a whim.

The Marshmallow Test is a classic research study performed at Stanford by behavioural scientist Walter Michel in the 1960s and 1970s. During the experiment, children are shown a marshmallow and told they can eat it now if they like. However, they can have two marshmallows if they wait a short time. Some children scoop up the marshmallow, while others resist.

According to Michel study, adults who had shown self-control as children performed better in school earned more money and were generally happier and more successful than those who did not resist the allure of the single marshmallow.

Steve Jobs is one of the most successful people in the world. When he searched for some idea, he would be so engrossed in the task that nothing else would matter to him. He could spend periods searching for new ideas at any cost. Steve Jobs says that work is a significant part of your life. You can do great work only if you love your work and are fully

> During the experiment, children are shown a marshmallow and told they can eat it now if they like. However, they can have two marshmallows if they wait a short time. Some children scoop up the marshmallow, while others resist.

"

What is the connection
between flow and
success, and how does
it facilitate it?

"

DNA

involved. It can be said about all these intelligent people of modern history that they laid the foundation of new creations by mobilising intuitive thinking with their logic.

The principle of success in this world depends on how creative and productive you are mentally and physically in your life. Success in today's world depends on how much knowledge you have in your profession and how much knowledge you have acquired. How much wealth and money did you earn, and what is your social status? And we see that behind all these successes, there is a need for an intelligent and creative mind.

> The **principle of success** in this **world depends on** how creative and **productive** you are mentally and **physically** in your **life.**

The key to success is to do great things as quickly as possible in your life. This is only possible when your focus and concentration are powerful and intense. With the help of the flow state, you can also gain the skills already attained by the world's most successful leaders and businesspeople. The flow state is the secret and the way through which you can concentrate all of the energies of your mind at one point.

The world's most successful people make positive changes in their minds through a flow state. Through this, they amply their abilities to solve problems. And this flow state multiplies the energies of their minds. The world's richest man, the founder of the Amazon company, recently surpassed Bill Gates in terms of wealth. His fortune is now estimated at 130 billion dollars. He started his company with an elementary idea. And that was to sell books online. He planned two to three years using the flow state instead of remaining in the present. This way, he left behind all of his opponents.

The key to success is ......

The key to
success is to do
great things as
quickly as
possible in your
life. This is
only possible
when your focus
and
concentration
are
powerful and
intense.

DNA

Step 4

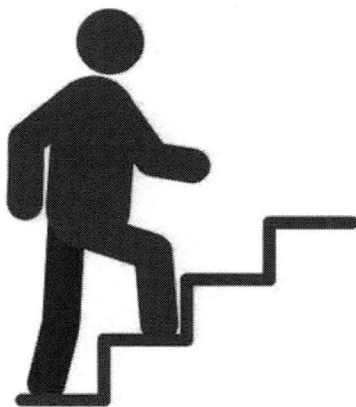

Here is a message from the Free Climbers sharing their successful strategies. A look at who they are and what we can learn from them?

In next few pages
you're about to find out!

- Those who climb mountains on their own without any assistance. They send a message that you should pay attention to !

- If you take every step of Life as if it guarantees your survival, you will give the utmost importance to every step of your Life.

- What is the best way to reach the top of your Life?

- How can deep focus be achieved?

There is a sport known as free climbing. Free climbers are different from traditional climbers. The climbers do not use ropes and do not rely on support. There is no hammer or nail with which they can climb the mountain. In the event of a mistake, a free climber does not have the safety measures that regular climbers do, which would prevent them from falling.

Climbing is not just a physical activity; it also requires a paradigm shift in how you approach and view of life. It tells us to focus on the possibilities rather than the obstacles. Take calculated risks, and don't be afraid to fail. Free climbers tell us that we must focus on what we can do instead of what we can't do. They need to be able to look at a seemingly impossible route and figure out how to make it possible. They must also trust their instincts and focus by gaining flow states.

Before climbing a mountain, a climber observes the peak and determines the direction of the peak to know where he is heading. As he climbs along these mountain paths, he becomes engrossed in them. Then, he forgets what direction the peak is facing and what direction the ground is. Let me give you an example. Before them, there is no room for error. For example, if they have to climb to an altitude of five thousand meters and have reached two thousand meters, then they have the peak above and the ground below. They are caught in the middle. If they make the wrong move, they

> **Climbing is not just a physical activity; it also requires a paradigm shift in how you approach and view of life. It tells us to focus on the possibilities rather than the obstacles.**

"

If you take every step
of life as if it
guarantees your
survival, you will
give the utmost
importance to every
step of your life.

"

DNA

could fall. They ascend towards the peak in this dangerous situation.

Research has revealed that these individuals are in a state of flow. In the very present moment, the focus is solely on their step. Their attention is devoted to the steps they are taking to ascend.

Neither are they considering the previous or the next step; they are concentrating solely on the present action, which is of primary importance. This step determines their fate. Therefore, they are neither afraid of falling nor excited about ascending. The purpose of this step at this stage is to ensure that it is complete and error-free as possible.

The very fact that they take this step is a guarantee of their survival. Therefore, they devote all of their attention to it.

They cut themselves off from the outside world and from time. To attain the flow state, they detached themselves from time and place and even from themselves.

> **Research** has revealed **that** these individuals are in a **state** of **flow.** In the present **moment,** the focus is **solely** on their **step.** **Their** attention is **devoted** to the **steps** they are **taking** to ascend.

To understand the flow state, you must decide your goal or what to achieve. Then, disregard the plan itself and concentrate solely on the steps, and the steps should be the focus of your attention. Having such a strong focus would be best if you could completely dissociate yourself from time and space.

To understand the flow state ......

To understand
the flow state,
you must
decide your
goal or what to
achieve. Then,
disregard the
plan itself and
concentrate
solely on the
steps, and the
steps should be
the focus
of your
attention.

DNA

Step 5

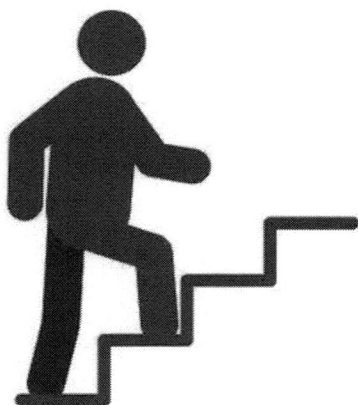

Identifying the most successful players' minds

In next few pages you're about to find out!

- How can a flow state break through comfort zone barriers?

- How did this man climb Mount Everest wearing shorts in extreme cold? You also have that power.

- Let us learn about Usain Bolt's journey to becoming one of the best athletes in the world. He achieved this feat by relentlessly pushing his flow state to new limits.

- How to overcome the fear of winning and losing? How best athletes and players do this to achieve the best performance by doing that. What we can Learn?

- What do great players Like Bradman and Tiger Wood have in common?

Ravizza was one of the first sports psychologists to describe how athletes felt at the peak of their performance. Based on interviews conducted with male and female athletes who played 12 different sports, the following characteristics were discovered:

Fear of failure could not keep them away from achieving their goals. They perform without much thinking. All the peak performers focus on one thing: they perform without effort. They have strong feeling of being in control. With disconnection of time and space. For them time is usually slowed down. They perceive the universe as integrated and unified experience. All of this is achieved by the Flow State

There is a very intense sport called Iron Man. The participants have to swim for 7 miles. Then they must ride a bicycle for 336 miles. This is followed by running for 78.6 miles. And all of these tasks have to be performed without rest and sleep. Such an intense task can only be achieved by attaining a flow state of mind. Christopher Herbergland claims that he had been made to perform this task by some universal power, which filled my joints and bones with energy.

Such extremely intense sports requiring a lot of steady and energetic flow to succeed need neurochemicals that can change the whole body and mind. It will make the mind so powerful that its energy can flow from the mind to every part of the body, and this is only possible through a flow state of mind.

Ravizza was one of the first sports psychologists to describe how athletes felt at the peak of their performance Based on interviews conducted with male and female athletes who played 12 different sports

No Longer fear of......

No Longer fear of
failure keeps us
from achieving our
goals. Perform
without thinking
Immersion at the
moment.
Focus on one thing:
performance without
effort. The feeling
of being in control.
Disconnection of
time and space
(usually slowed
down)

DNA

"

How can a flow state break through comfort zone barriers?

DNA

"

Wim Hof, also known as Iceman, is 49 years old. He is a resident of Holland. He has made 12 world records; no other person can make it. He has climbed Mount Everest naked, wearing only shorts and knickers. He has also climbed Africa's tallest, Mount Kilimanjaro. This man has run barefoot on the Finnish ice cliffs at minus 32 degrees for 26 miles wearing shorts and has done it without taking any respite.

> He has also climbed Africa's tallest, Mount Kilimanjaro. This man has run barefoot on the Finnish ice cliffs at minus 32 degrees for 26 miles wearing a knicker and has done it without taking any respite.

Scientists are researching his brain. It seems he descends into a flow state of mind, making his body and mind irrelevant to the external challenges and the adverse effects of cold weather outside. Some parts of his brain stimulate neurochemicals when he attains a flow state. For example, opioids and cannabinoids eliminate his pain. Then the parts of the brain successfully release dopamine and serotonin, which becomes a cause of peace and contentment. And it is these chemicals that strengthen his belief that he can achieve even the most challenging goal.

Usain Bolt is the first-ever athlete in history, who won three gold medals in 100 meters race in the Olympics. When he landed for the third time in the 100-meter race, the TV cameras in the stadium first showed the faces of the other seven contestants, and all of their faces were serious. Usain Bolt had a smile on his face when the cameras showed him. When the 100-meter race started, Justin Gatlin was ahead of Usain Bolt. With about 40 meters left, Usain Bolt leaves everyone behind one by one.

The world saw that he had left everyone behind as if he were

"

Let us learn about Usain Bolt's journey to becoming one of the best athletes in the world. He achieved this feat by relentlessly pushing his flow state to new limits.

"

DNA

running on water, not land. He had become a great athlete in the world. He was not afraid of losing from the beginning. He had transcended defeat and victory, millions of people sitting in the stadium, the TV cameras, and his opponents, and he had sunk into the sea of his performance. We call this flow state.

The difference between his brain and his opponents' brains is that he could convert the brain's simple Beta waves into extraordinary electrical brain waves, namely Alpha and Theta electric waves. The special cocktail of neurochemicals had been prepared in his brain, amplified his mental and physical powers, and became the guarantor of his success.

> The **difference** between his **brain** and his **opponents'** brains is that he could **convert** the **brain's simple** Beta **waves** into extraordinary **electrical** brain **waves**, namely **Alpha and Theta**

The psychological research done in the world of sports shows whether it is Don Bradman's triple century, Michael Jordan's basketball shot, or Tiger Woods's golf shots. The superpower flow state of mind has always been involved in high performance. People get so busy with their action that the activity goes on automatically. They stop being aware of themselves as being detached from the actions they are performing.

There are two reasons why flow is associated with better performance, according to Engeser and Rheinberg (2008). The first benefit of flow is that it is a highly functional state that should be able to increase performance. It has been shown that individuals who experience flow often have better motivation to continue performing further activities. This leads them to set themselves more challenging tasks to experience flow again. Thus, flow can be seen as a motivational force that motivates us to achieve excellence.

Due to this, there is a higher level of concentration on the task at hand. Additionally, there is also a loss of self and increased mental

capabilities allowing players and athletes to become more efficient
& effective.

There is also a loss of self ......

Due to this,
there is a higher
level of
concentration on
the task at hand.
Additionally,
there is also a
loss of self and
increased mental
capabilities
allowing players
and athletes to
become more
efficient &
effective.

DNA

Step 6

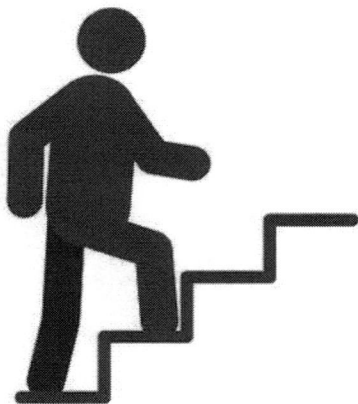

Is there a brain king who rules us?

Discovering the hidden intelligence that has been suppressed and how to regain it

In next few pages you're about to find out!

- What is the part of our brain that governs the mind? And keeps us in a logical box. How freedom from this is possible?

- Due to the dictator of this brain, many intelligent areas of our mind are under control. How to free these intelligent areas of our brain?

- One secret you should know: intelligence exists in many other areas and places in the brain.

- How the great genius scientist, poets, and thinkers defeats this dictator of his mind

- After flow waves silences the prefrontal cortex's rule, the suppressed intelligence areas will become independent

L et me tell you an exciting thing about the function of the brain here. If you know this secret, you can create great and unique thoughts in your life. And you can make such decisions based on these new and unique thoughts, which will increase the performance of your life.

Successful people have used super-logical thinking for their success and creations. Their ability to break complex ideas into smaller components made them uniquely successful. They then use this to analyse a problem, develop creative solutions and make the right decisions. This helps them to move closer to their ultimate goals at super speed.

My research has led to some interesting facts based on various articles and research papers. Let me explain it to you in simple terms about the flow state. Who rules our brains? When we are involved in our daily routines, the waves running on the surface of our brain during that cannot create great thoughts and ideas. The area that governs is the prefrontal cortex of the brain frontal lobe. This part of the brain determines the selection of subject, topic and train of our thoughts. It is the part where the logical debate occurs.

This is the part of our brain called the logical brain that is in charge of rational thinking, reasoning, and

The function of the brain here. If you know this secret, you can create great and unique thoughts in your life. And you can make such decisions based on these new and unique thoughts

"

What is the part of
our brain that
governs the mind?
And keeps us in a
logical box. How is
freedom from this
possible?

"

DNA

decision-making. This is where all the information is tested, and the opinions we form based on this information are also conceived in this area. If we consider the mind as a country or like a kingdom, the prefrontal cortex is the ruling dictator. It rules our brains. But there is a compulsion and limitation of this area that this part of the brain depends only on the available limited information and cannot think out of the box.

One more secret you should know: intelligence exists in many other areas and places in the brain. The prefrontal cortex, the king of our mind, does not allow these brain centers to give their opinions and maintains its dictatorship. Some powerful electric waves are generated during the flow state, which silences this dictator and ruler of our minds.

> **This is where all** the information **is tested,** and the **opinions we form based on this** information **are also** conceived in **this area.**

After flow waves silence the prefrontal cortex's rule, the suppressed intelligence areas are now independent. These areas are now free to give their brilliant opinions to our minds. These liberated areas of intelligence provide us with unique ideas, and the fantastic thing about them is that they can think out of the box. It is this unique method of thinking through which the most successful people create new and unique ideas and creations.

When in the 'State of Flow', time slows down in the inner world and speeds up in the outer world. The inside world reappears for us, and the outside world disappears. In order to explain why all of this happens, we need to understand that our brain's master controller, the pre-frontal cortex, is put to sleep while we are awake. When this area is quietened during the flow state, our instinctive brain begins to awaken, allowing us to make decisions and act based on

One more secret intelligence
exists in......

One more
secret intelligence
exists in many
other areas and
places in the brain.
The prefrontal
cortex, the king of
our mind,
does not allow
these brain
centres to give
their opinions and
maintains its
dictatorship

DNA

"

What is the secret of
the neuroscience
behind the rule of
this dictator of the
mind and the
unnecessary logical
pressure making us
fail?

"

DNA

instinct rather than reason.

In my opinion, there is a supra-logic tracks embedded in our minds, but we are not able to identify it. In terms of innovation and solving a problem, the flow state leaps straight from the problem to the solution without running through any recurring thoughts.

In order to succeed, you must be able to think innovatively and intelligently. In order to be intelligent and innovative, we need to think outside the box." However, the problem with this is that we are creatures of habit. We are most comfortable in our familiar routines of thinking.

This book will convince you that thinking beyond the box is one of the most valuable skills that anyone can learn. Flow state can be referred to as the thread that ties together two disparate ideas, which is the essence of originality and innovation.

> **When in the 'State of Flow', time slows down in the inner world and speeds up in the outer world. disappears**

This book will convince you ......

This book
will convince you
that thinking
beyond the box is
one of the most
valuable skills
that anyone can
learn. Flow state
can be referred
to as the thread
that ties together
two disparate
ideas, which is the
essence of
originality and
innovation

DNA

Step 7

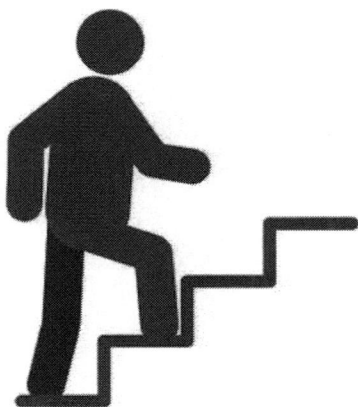

Your brain works like a radio, learn and hack it

In next few pages
you're about to find out!

- It may surprise you that the brain is also an electrical machine. It uses electrical signals to communicate with the rest of the body. These signals allow us to think, move, feel, and remember.

- How can high-quality electrical currents and electrical waves work best for brain? To ensure proper electrical currents, what do we need to do?

- How do brain surface waves affect the brain in terms of its function?

- The way the brain selects its channels is like how a radio selects its channels.

- Brain surface waves are rhythmic patterns of electrical activity produced by neurons in the brain. These waves help the brain to select the most relevant signals. How to get the best wave and best current?

Electricity is present everywhere, even within the human body. The human body is powered by electric currents that operate at a very low voltage. Brain is also an electrical organ powered and operated by electric current flowing in the form of waves. Movement, thinking, and feeling is possible because of electricity, which transmits signals throughout the body and to the brain.

The average neuron is estimated to have a resting voltage of around 70 microvolts or 0.07 volts at rest. Comparatively, this is quite a low voltage when compared to 1.5 volts found in a standard AA battery. It is through electrical impulses, called brain waves that the cells in the brain communicate with each other. As it is necessary to have a high-quality voltage in an electronic instrument, the same is true for a high-quality electrical current and appropriate wave are needed for brain to work at its best.

You'll understand the methods of thinking and its foundations when you have a good understanding of how the brain works. Let's take this analogy the brain works like a radio set.

We know the radio set has a receiver antenna that receives channels. What's being received are radio frequency waves sent by the radio station. This receiver gets the radio's transmissions. As a matter of fact, this is how our brain functions. Let me give you a little background to

> Brain, is also an electrical organ powered and operated by electric current flowing in the form of waves. Movement, thinking and feeling are possible

You'll understand the ......

You'll
understand the
matter of
thinking and its
foundations when
you have a good
understanding
of how
the brain
works.

DNA

"

How can high-quality electrical currents and electrical waves work best? To ensure proper electrical currents, what do we need to do?

"

DNA

understand what I am trying to explain. In addition to the receiver, there is a knob on the radio set. If we turn it, we will be able to select the different channels that we wish to listen to.

Simply turn the knob on the radio , and you can choose the channel you wish to listen to. The same is true for the brain model. The brain also has some receivers that can receive different kinds of information, such as thinking topic channels.

Adjusting the knob of a radio set selects the channels of the radio set. This knob of the brain is responsible for selecting the topics we think about.is called the prefrontal cortex. Prefrontal cortex is a part of frontal lobe above our eyes. This part of the brain is essential for higher-level thinking, decision-making, and problem-solving. The prefrontal cortex is responsible for helping us to think about the topics we choose to focus on.

Simply, turn the and you can **choose** and **adjust** the **channel** you wish to **Listen** to. The **same** is **true** for the brain **model.** The **brain** also **has** some receivers **that** can **receive** different **kinds** of **information**

There is another interesting fact you should be aware of, as a radio set is an electrical instrument, so is the brain, it is an electrical organ. The brain, to function correctly, needs frequencies of electrical waves, just as a radio set requires frequencies of radio waves. This is why it is imperative to understand that the frequencies the brain needs can be tailored to an individual's needs. These frequencies can be altered through the various exercises and methods described in this book. By understanding and altering the energy frequencies the brain needs, we can ensure that our brains are functioning optimally.

The brain to function
correctly needs ......

As a radio set is
an electrical
instrument, so is
the brain, which
is an electrical
organ. The
brain, to
function
correctly, needs
frequencies of
energy, just as a
radio set
requires
frequencies of
radio waves.

DNA

Step 8

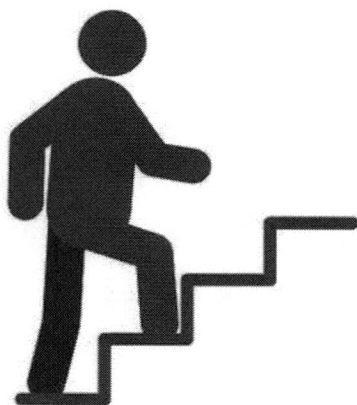

Learn the brain's simple language and become a better thinker

In next few pages
you're about to find out!

- What is the mechanism by which brain regions and cells communicate? Here's a simple explanation

- What are the brain's languages? How can you understand it and increase your brain language power easily?

- What brain chemical plays a fundamental role in every process, from happiness to sadness and intelligence to discovery?

- What chemical cocktail does the brain need most? How can you make it at any age?

- Precious molecules and chemicals in your brain are made every day, but you throw them away. How can they be used?

- To succeed in life, which Brain Language should you use?

- In your brain, what are the most precious electrical waves?

- What is the process by which cannabis-like chemicals are released in the brain, and how can they be used?

- What is the chemical that turns off your fear and defeat switch so that you are no longer afraid of losing?

Learn what language your Brain speaks – How to master them. In my opinion, the Brain has two types of languages, electrical and chemical. To understand both languages of the Brain, we must understand brain cells. These brain cells are called neurons. Typically, neurons have a structure called a body, and a rope-like structure called an axon.

It is important to note that brain cells are always active. Their activity is also known as neuronal firing. To better understand this phenomenon, let me give you an example. In the same way that you have probably seen stars shining, I want to make it easier for you to understand that brain cells behave like stars and shine like stars.

As stars shine due to electrical and chemical processes, brain cells also function because of electrical and chemical processes. A neuronal firing will result in electrical waves that create an electric current in the Brain.

These electrical waves are known as brain waves. In the case of neurons, they travel out of their bodies and into the axons of neurons, which are the wires that transmit information from one brain cell to another. Brain waves have many effects and are believed to influence all brain functions in various ways.

In my opinion, the Brain has two types of Languages, electrical and chemical. To understand both Languages of the Brain, we must understand its brain cells

The fact that we now understand that the number of times a neuron shines or is active during a specific period will determine the number of brain waves produced by that neuron. If a neuron flashes fifteen times a second, the same number of waves will be produced in the same time frame. Furthermore, a neuron that sparks fifty times will generate fifty waves in the same amount of time. In scientific terms, this is also known as frequency.

A brain cell has doors on its body surface, similar to a door in a house, and, like a large house, a brain cell can have many doors on its surface. Open doors allow various chemicals to enter and exit the Brain cells, that is, the neurons, depending on the chemicals they contain. In the same way as when a person opens a door, they can come in and go out of the house, just as when a brain wave opens a door on a brain cell, chemicals can also enter and leave the cell in the same manner. In neuroscience, we refer to these doors as channels into the Brain and the chemicals that enter and leave the brain cells as neurotransmitters.

The function of these neurotransmitters is to regulate the electrical activity of brain cells. The brain wave is formed because of the electrical activity that occurs within the brain tissue. Different types of brain waves can be classified in the following ways: They are referred to as five different types of electrical waves based on the frequency at which they occur in the Brain.

Your Brain has five different types of waves. Brain waves, each of which operates at a different speed.

> **The fact** that we now understand that the **number** of times a neuron **shines or is** active **during** a specific **period** will determine the **number** of brain **waves**

A brain cell has ......

A brain cell has doors on its body surface, similar to a door in a house, and, like a large house, a brain cell can have many doors on its surface. Open doors allow various chemicals to enter and exit the Brain, that is, the neurons, depending on the chemicals they contain

DNA

From the fastest to the slowest, five different types of brain waves include:

- Gamma
- Beta
- Alpha
- Theta
- Delta

Beta waves occur when the Brain works on goal-oriented tasks, such as planning a meeting or actively reflecting on a particular issue. Being alert, attentive and engaged in day-to-day challenges results from being engaged in 'fast' activities. These waves are not the best for bringing forth new intelligent and innovative ideas. The result is that Brain is forced to perform at a significantly lower level than its exciting potential and capabilities.

Beta waves are of great importance for reacting and making day-to-day decisions. Still, Alpha waves are vital for absorbing information, maintaining alertness while remaining calm, integrating mind and body, and picking up new skills. Alpha waves are slower than Beta waves, and Theta waves are slower than Alpha waves. All these brain waves represent a more powerful electric environment for optimal Brain functioning in certain situations, such as in deep concentration.

Alpha waves are vital for absorbing information, maintaining alertness while remaining calm, integrating mind and body, and picking up new skills.

All these slower waves on the Brain can create flow state magic. Deep divine synergy can be achieved by implementing this electrochemical model of the Brain.

Here is a simple answer for those wondering what can be done then. One can enter a flow state by altering our brain wave patterns or adjusting our neurons' firing rate and frequency. The Flow State was reached by converting the beta waves into alpha waves or slower brain waves.

The following chapters will describe various methods and means to generate these valuable waves regularly in our busy daily lives. The Brain produces certain chemicals when electric waves are generated, causing the brain cells to release them. A message is sent from one cell to another by these chemicals. Let's talk about these chemicals in the next chapter.

Alpha waves are slower than ......

Alpha waves are
slower than Beta
waves, and Theta
waves are slower
than Alpha waves.
All these brain
waves represent a
more powerful
electric environment
for optimal Brain
functioning in
certain situations,
such as in deep
concentration.

DNA

Step 9

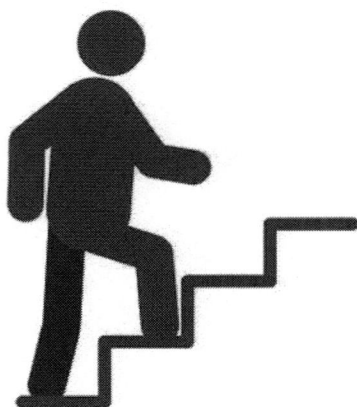

Here are your most powerful brain chemicals. Find out which cocktail is the best and how to get it?

In next few pages
you're about to find out!

- During flow states, which neurochemicals serve as cement for rebuilding your brain?

- You can create and use superfast mind tracks when these brain-produced chemicals are released during flow.

- Dopamine causes your success, and it is the one brain chemical which can cause your failure.

- Let me introduce you to a very interesting chemical that you have in your brain, Anandamide.

The word is derived from the
Sanskrit term "Ananda", which
means "bliss".

- Engaging in a flow state
  increases Dopamine naturally and
  promotes the release of the finest
  blend of chemicals

- This also answers an intriguing
  question I have had in my mind for
  years. Now I know why a painter,
  a poet or a philosopher becomes
  addicted to their work

It would be most beneficial if you had the most nourishing cocktail of chemicals for idea generation, innovative thinking and clever decisions. It would help to have a delicate balance of these precious chemical pearls in your brain.

Flow state spells in the brain must be repeated to produce an enriching combination of chemicals. You can create and use superfast mind tracks when these brain-produced chemicals are released during flow. This chemical combination also helps to increase the speed of thought processes and the ability to learn, retain and retrieve more information.

Therefore, different types of intelligence arise when there is more grey matter - more neuronal connections - in specific brain regions associated with things referred to as 'brainier, Ingredients. This additional grey matter makes it possible for the brain to form more complex connections that enable it to think more sophisticatedly. It also allows for more efficient storage and retrieval of information, allowing people to draw on a larger pool of knowledge to come up with innovative solutions to problems.

Neurochemicals are those chemical compounds of the brain which have different types. Among these is the most powerful weapon of your mind, which is known as Dopamine.

> **Flow state** spells in the **brain** must be repeated to **produce** an **enriching** combination of **chemicals.** You can create and use **superfast** mind tracks **when** these brain-produced **chemicals** are released during **flow**

"

During flow states,
which neurochemicals
serve as cement for
rebuilding your
brain?
"

DNA

Dopamine is a neurochemical that you can compare with pearls. This is the pearl of intelligence produced almost every day in your brain. But it would be best if you used it correctly. It performs essential functions in the brain for you. Dopamine causes your success, and it is the one brain chemical which can cause your failure. It all depends on where and in which part of your brain it is used and for which activity. Creative activity or just a pleasure-seeking activity. It is your choice. The most promising chemical of the brain you need to be successful.

> **Dopamine causes your success, and it is the one brain chemical which can cause your failure**

There is no doubt that Dopamine plays a crucial role in how we feel. In my view, it's one of the most integral aspects of our unique ability to plan and think. We all need higher quality and quantity of thoughts in our brains at the right place and time. This makes things more interesting, leads us to work harder, and makes us pay attention to details.

The other important neurotransmitter along with dopamine is epinephrine They both work together to increase your concentration and stream your body with feel-good sensations which reward you for your increased focus and your enhanced concentration.

Let me introduce you to a very interesting chemical that you have in your brain, Anandamide. The word is derived from the Sanskrit term "Ananda", which means "bliss". Basically, it is a neurotransmitter that functions through the cannabinoids in the human nervous system. These chemicals of your brain turn off the fear centre, the Amygdala, and hence there is less fear and anxiety.

Dopamine is a neurochemical ......

Dopamine is a neurochemical or neurotransmitter that you can compare with pearls. This is the pearl of intelligence produced almost every day in your brain. But it would be best if you used it correctly. It performs essential functions in the brain for you. What are its functions?

DNA

"

Dopamine causes your success, and it is the one brain chemical which can cause your failure.
"

DNA

Our third friend in the mix is serotonin. It is believed that it shows up at the tail end of the flow and gives us the feeling of peace and tranquillity after experiencing flow.

Engaging in a flow state increases Dopamine naturally and promotes the release of the finest blend of chemicals. Anandamide stimulates lateral thinking, and endorphins modulate stress levels by keeping your calm.

Engaging in a flow state increases **Dopamine** naturally and **promotes** the **release** of the finest blend of **chemicals**

To give you the perspective, The most addictive drug gives it a score of 3 out of a maximum score of 3. Heroin is an opiate that causes the level of Dopamine in the brain's reward system to increase by up to 200% in experimental animals. Considering what I just said, you can see why I meant flow states are powerful; it is because attaining flow states of mind is like taking a small amount of cocaine, heroin, and anti-depressants simultaneously! This is a natural method for thinkers and geniuses to get a chemical boost in their thinking.

Eureka, I found an answer to a question that I had in my mind for a very long time, at least for many years. I was wondering why creative people became addicted to creativity and discoveries. Why could painters spend hours and hours painting, poets' dwell in deep thoughts, and scientists forget time connectivity while working on their theories? The answer is that they are getting cannabis-like chemicals released in their minds resulting in a blissful state. Now I understand why this process is so addictive and rewarding for creative minds. They can experience joy and satisfaction from the process and feel accomplished and deeply fulfilled. Unsurprisingly, they develop a habit that is an addiction to working and repeatedly getting into the flow zone.

Considering what I just said ......

Considering what I
just said, you
can see why I
meant flow states are
powerful; it is because
attaining flow states
of mind is like taking
cocaine, heroin, and
anti-depressants
simultaneously! This is
a natural method for
thinkers and geniuses
to get a chemical
boost in their thinking.

DNA

Step 10

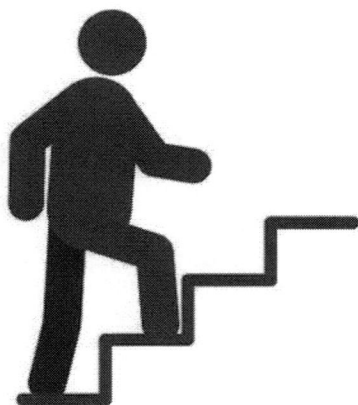

The brain area that controls our emotions and how flow states create a state of heightened creativity and focus?

In next few pages you're about to find out!

- Where is the emotion King in our brain?

- How does the Limbic system control our emotions? Let's find out.

- How can we produce chemicals like cannabis that give us blissful moments in our brains? How does the flow state protect us from anxiety?

To answer the question, 'Who is the king of all emotions in our minds?' We must discover one fundamental fact about ourselves. It is the limbic system, which that regulates our emotions. The limbic system is responsible for the production of chemicals that influence our emotions, and it is also the area of the brain that processes and stores memories. It plays an important role in our emotional well-being, and it is the king of all emotions in our minds.

Embedded deep within the brain is a complex network of interconnected brain structures. A part of the human brain called the amygdale plays a vital role in handling strong emotions, such as fear or pleasure.

A flow state can play a huge role in generating an electrochemical environment to calm your king of emotions, which is the amygdala, to generate emotions of bliss. This blissful state is key to calming the mind and reducing stress. Another interesting aspect of flow states is that you are working, but you are doing it in a different way from others.

In contrast to others, you're fully immersed, allowing you to experience a blissful state of mind. With this feeling of contentment, a flow state can help treat anxiety and depression by providing an environment to relax the mind and body. This allows individuals to have a different perspective on their emotions.

> **A flow state can play a huge role in generating an electrochemical environment to calm your king of emotions, which is the amygdala, to generate emotions of bliss.**

"

How does the Limbic
system control our
emotions? Let's find
out.

DNA　　　"

As we proceed along the flowing journey, this process helps us maintain a sense of meaning, hope, and fulfilment.

The development of flow states leads to a change in the perception of the passage of time. As time slows, the sense of urgency diminishes, which ultimately contributes to the reduction of anxiety levels.

During a state of flow, people can experience autotelic phenomena, which can make them happy no matter where they are, whether on a desert island or in confinement. Unlike most people, they don't succumb to the unbearable conditions they face because they transform them into manageable and even pleasurable struggles.

> During a state of flow, people can experience autotelic phenomena, which can make them happy no matter where they are, whether on a desert island or in confinement.

In my opinion, the best moments in our lives are led by flow because the body or mind of a person is stretched to the limit in a voluntary effort to accomplish something difficult but worthwhile." During this time, the electrical waves calm our emotional king, the amygdala. Various chemical cocktails, such as cannabinoids, have been created to neutralize the fear factors to make people less afraid of the unknown.

The ability to repeat creative thoughts or actions which you enjoy is essential for activating flow. When you succeed in creating a result, no matter what it may be, your brain is flooded with dopamine. The feel-good chemical helps motivate you as you accomplish your goal. The dopamine hit you receive after being in the flow will influence you toward similar behaviour

"

How can we produce
chemicals like
cannabis that give us
blissful moments in
our brains? How does
the flow state
protect us from
anxiety?

"

DNA

The development of
flow states ......

The
development
of flow states
leads to
a change in the
perception
of the passage
of time.
As time slows,
the sense
of urgency
diminishes which
ultimately contributes
to the reduction of
anxiety levels.

DNA

Step 11

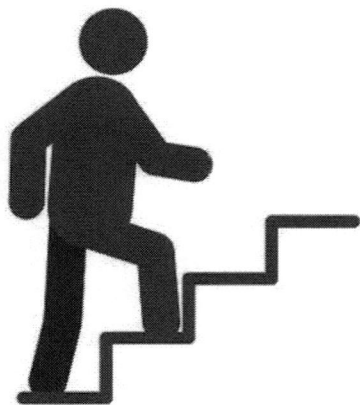

The best way to come up with ideas without overthinking

In next few pages you're about to find out!

- Ideas are like dreams. How do they come about? Your thinking perception will never be the same after you hear my hypothesis.

- It is estimated that there are seventy thousand thoughts in a day, but what if there was even one idea?

- The best ideas can come to you like dreams during waking hours. Learn the technique.

- When you sleep, do you construct your dreams? What will we learn from the answer to this question?

- How is it possible to generate ideas, the highest thoughts, in one's mind without overthinking them?

- Suppose a situation in which, in front of your eyes, a building and its walls were created automatically without a single worker being present. Can the buildings of creation in your mind be built like that?

- Great ideas and general thoughts - what is the difference? Nothing can stop you from succeeding if you know this.

An exciting aspect of a flow state is that once you are in it, you do not have to think as much to generate ideas or learn. There would be a magical phenomenon that would occur as brilliant ideas would begin to appear on the screen of your mind. It is similar to dreams that appear on your mind's screen without you thinking or creating them.

Please allow me to give you some straightforward examples to help you better understand the ideas and change your thoughts. Flow State of mind is a mysterious and unique phenomenon that can trigger ideas like dreams. To illustrate, let me give you an example of dreaming while you are sleeping.

It is natural to dream while sleeping. Everyone understands this. Dreaming is nothing unusual. So here is my question for you. The question is, have you ever wondered if the dream you had last night was yours? The answer is, of course, yes. The dream appeared in my mind. I saw it in my head. Did you create this dream, or were you compelled to do so? Did it come to you spontaneously? while you were sleeping. The answer to all these questions is a loud resounding yes.

This is my point, which explains the concept of ideas arising in the flow state of mind. Indeed, ideas occur like a flash of a dream. Although you are not overthinking the concept, you are not

> There would be a magical phenomenon that would occur as brilliant ideas would begin to appear on the screen of your mind. It is similar to dreams that appear on your mind's screen without you thinking or creating them.

deliberately creating it, yet it appears to you when your mind reaches a state of flow.

Unsurprisingly, brilliant ideas are conceived when average thoughts are stitched together. It links a simple thought with another simple thought and these two with a third thought. This process may also be referred to as the flow led semi-conscious flashing of ideas. As during sleep, you did not create your dream, your mind did it for you without you having any major conscious control. Similarly, in flow state, ideas are created for you by your mind without you having a major conscious control.

It would be interesting to see if, after a period of time, the bricks start aligning spontaneously on top of each other without the assistance of labourers.

Please keep an open mind that it is more likely that you will start developing a new idea once your original one has been clearly defined. In my experience, creative and intelligent minds generate original ideas in this manner. Combining simple but straightforward thoughts makes it possible to develop a unique idea due to synthesising super activity in the flow state.

Let me give you an example. Workers are employed to complete the project when a building is being constructed. To complete the construction, one brick is placed on the second brick and the other on the third brick. Consider your thoughts as bricks. As soon as you enter a flow state, you initially consciously place bricks of thought on each other, one after the other.

It would be interesting to see if, after a period of time, the bricks start aligning spontaneously on top of each other without the assistance of labourers. Then they start to have a life of their own. This is precisely what happens when you enter Flow State. After some time, the bricks, that is, these thoughts, begin to form a structure. It's like a building is being built inside your head on its own.

Unsurprisingly, brilliant ideas ......

Unsurprisingly, brilliant ideas are conceived when average thoughts are stitched together. It links a simple thought with another simple thought and these two with a third thought. This process may also be referred to as the generation of flash ideas.

DNA

"

When you sleep, do
you construct your
dreams? What will
we learn from the
answer to this
question?

"

DNA

This can be understood through another example. Driverless cars are a concept that is becoming more and more popular. Vehicles that don't require a driver to operate them are referred to as self-driving vehicles. Using sensors, they control their direction and speed based on the information they receive from these sensors.

Please understand that this is a picture of your mind's appearance after coming to the flow state. It becomes necessary to start the car of thoughts at some point, but once it is started, it will run automatically. Similarly, it would help if you read more about the topic on which you seek inspiration. When you spend time connecting a subject to a target, you will find that it becomes second nature. It is when you concentrate on a particular topic continuously. As a result, you will surely come up with new ideas that will surprise you.

This intense focus allows ......

This intense
focus allows you
to absorb and
retain more
information and
make better
decisions,
making you
more productive
and successful.

DNA

Step 12

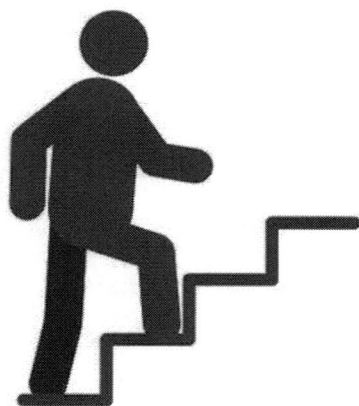

Identify the target, then forget it and focus on the steps that will lead there- Japanese philosophy

In next few pages you're about to find out!

- How to aim accurately even with a blindfold, a Japanese principle?

- After setting the target, why should it be forgotten? An important secret

- Know when a step becomes more valuable than a destination.

- Why is it important to master the steps leading up to the goal?

German professor Eugene Hazel was transferred to Japan in 1920. He had come to Tokyo University to teach philosophy. A few years later, the professor decided to learn Japanese martial arts and archery to better understand Japanese culture. To learn the basics of archery, he went to Ava Kenzo, one of the most excellent archers of the time.

During his beginner classes on archery, he was mentored by the great teacher Awa Kenzo. Initially, the grandmaster Awa Kenzo instructed him to learn the fundamentals. In order to learn this basic skill, Professor Herrigel had to put in a lot of time and effort. To the grandmaster, Herrigel complained that it was challenging to learn archery quickly.

Kenzo explained something insightful: measuring the path and counting time is not necessary to reach a goal. We do all our efforts no matter how long it takes, whether it takes days, months, or years. Despite efforts, Herrigel's performance was dismal when he was allowed to shoot at more distant targets. He became more discouraged with each shot that flew off course. Herrigel concluded that his poor aim must be the cause of his problems.

As Kenzo explained to his student, what matters is not how and what a person aims but how one approaches the target really matters. "You should be able to hit it blindfolded if the aim is unimportant," Herrigel yelled.

German professor Eugene Hazel was transferred to Japan in 1920. He had come to Tokyo University to teach philosophy. A few years later, the professor decided to learn Japanese martial arts and archery

Kenzo explained......

Kenzo
explained
something
insightful:
measuring
the path and
counting
time is not
necessary to
reach a
goal.

DNA

"

Why is it important to master the steps Leading up to the goal and mastering them?

"

DNA

Zero to Volcano - 33 Steps to Superstate of your Magical Mind
by DNA

Grand Master accepted the challenge and was taken to the practice hall that night, where the target was hidden in the dark. Once Kenzo had settled into his shooting stance, he tightened the bowstring and released the first arrow into the darkness towards the target being blindfolded.

The professor was surprised when he was able to see the arrow had hit its target. The arrow was skilfully attached to its mark and reflected the grand master's words. After setting a goal, not the actual goal, but the steps that need to be mastered to achieve the goal matter most. How much work have you done to achieve it, and for how many years have you pursued it? What is the position of your body when shooting an arrow? What is the direction of your eyes? What is the rate of your breathing? You need to master all these things to hit the target.

The important thing was to focus on the steps you must take and the steps you must learn to achieve your goal. The steps are more important than the goal itself. After setting a goal, not the actual goal itself, the steps that must be mastered to achieve it are important. There is a lesson in this story. After setting your goal, you should immerse yourself in the skill required to achieve this goal. You should be so involved that even if you aim blindfolded at your target, you can still hit the target. You can achieve the goal with precision and efficiency if you devote yourself to the steps required to master the skill.

After setting your goal ......

After setting
your goal, you
should immerse
yourself in the
skill required to
achieve this
goal.
You should
be so involved
that even if
you aim
blindfolded

DNA

Step 13

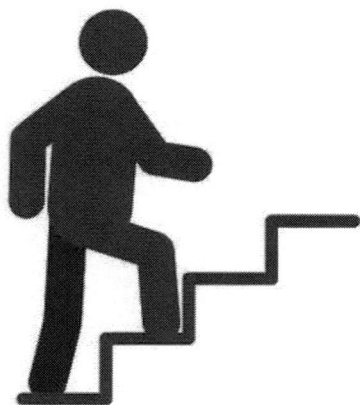

Identifying the single most important factor for success. Let's figure out the easiest way to focus

In next few pages
you're about to find out!

- What is the importance of focusing on focus? Make your success possible with research?

- Why is it important to pay attention to yourself?

- Why is your focus the most responsible for your success? A big revelation.

- Bird's Eye - a story from thousands of years and its hidden secret.

- Who will do it for you, if you, yourself wont?

You must pay attention to your attention because it is the gateway to your thinking, perception, memory, learning, reasoning, problem-solving, and decision-making. It would help if you thought effectively to produce the quality work necessary to succeed.

With a strong focus, all aspects of your thinking ability will be improved. Focus is enhanced by flow state waves. Flow state waves allow us to concentrate our energy and stay focused for longer periods of time, resulting in improved cognitive performance. Focusing on the flow state will greatly enhance your ability to think critically.

To make your work super effective, you must focus on the right things. If you can concentrate well, you will save time. Whenever you lose focus on your work your life output will be lower, and you will have to spend longer. In the absence of concentration, you cannot think effectively. You must think exceedingly well to produce the quality of work required to succeed.

Thus, it is easy to understand why focus is crucial to success. However, achieving deep focus can be challenging; not many people have this skill. We know the mind jumps from one thought to another every second, making it challenging to focus on just one stream of topic. Experts estimate that we have 60,000 to 80,000 thoughts per day. What would be the point if most of them were useless and pointless?

> **With a strong focus, all aspects of your thinking ability will be improved. Focus is enhanced by flow state waves.**

"

What is the
importance of
focusing on focus?
Make your success
possible with
research?

"

DNA

Experts estimate that......

Experts estimate that we have 60,000 to 80,000 thoughts per day. What would be the point if most of them were useless and pointless

DNA

"

What is the
importance of
focusing on focus?
Make your success
possible with
research?

"

DNA

There is a story about a Guru asking three disciples to shoot a bird's eye while sitting on a tree branch. The disciple who came first drew an arrow and aimed it at the bird. As the teacher asked the disciple, what do you see he replied and said, I can see the sky, a tree, a branch of the tree, and the bird sitting on the branch. The disciple who shot the arrow missed.

Then, the Guru called another disciple and ordered him to shoot at the bird's eye. The Guru again asked the other disciple the same question when he placed the arrow in the bow. The disciple replied that he could see the branch. The bird was visible sitting on it, and then he also aimed but missed the target when he shot the arrow.

> **Achieving** deep **focus** can be **challenging;** not **many** people **have this skill.** We know the **mind** jumps **from** one **thought** to another **every second**

Then he asked the third disciple to aim. After he had put the arrow in the bow and made the position, he asked him the same question. He replied that he could see nothing, only the bird's eye, and as soon as he fired the shot, he had hit the target. We find from this story that without an eagle's-eye view of our target, our target may not fall into place, and we may not achieve the goal in life that we are capable of.

A big question, a big secret, is why can't you focus? In your brain, there is no single point of focus. Oue focus is due to a vast network of brain regions that collectively make up your brain's "attention system" - a system that interacts closely with your thoughts, actions, and feelings to assist you in managing them more effectively.

Thousands of years ago, humans had to consider the past, present, and future simultaneously instead of trying to limit themselves entirely to the present. To assess the dangers in the environment. Throughout evolution, man has used the default thinking network for thousands of years. It is that network which shifts our thoughts from past to present to future so that we do not become oblivious to our dangers like the people of the Stone Age. The attack of a dinosaur or the attack of a bloodthirsty lion. One had to always remain vigilant to survive.

The same evolutionary process has been transmitted to the brain of a modern man, thousands of years later. This network is the biggest enemy of our focus, and it only lets us retain our focus for a short time. Hence, even today, it is difficult for a person to continue to work on a single task for a long time and for his mind to remain focused on just one subject.

This book will help you to go beyond this network and reach your hidden mental networking treasures.

We find from this story that without an eagle's-eye view of our target, our entire focus and attention, our target may not fall into place, and we may not achieve the goal in life that we are capable of

Slowly being taken away......

The flow state triggers
mind techniques and
formulas needed to
hit the target in Life.
Let me tell you
one thing: our
attention span and
focus are two of
our most
extraordinary
abilities, but
they are
slowly being
taken away.

DNA

Step 14

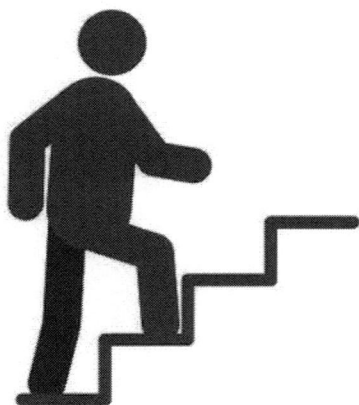

Explore the relationship between your thoughts and your focus of mind. What you can do to take control?

In next few pages you're about to find out!

- You're about to discover an exciting way to connect your thoughts, mind, and focus. There are endless possibilities.

- How do you expand the horizons of your mind?

- Are you looking to broaden your perspective and strengthen your relationship with yourself?

- All of us have a major sense of disbelief about ourselves.

searched with fascination for an example explaining the relationship between our mind and focus. I needed a simple illustration explaining the relationship between the mind and focus. What is the link between our thoughts and what we focus on?

The moment we start talking about this topic, most of us start feeling uncomfortable. This is because many think the mind is an arid and challenging subject. When we enter such a state, our thinking and understanding switches are shut down. Nevertheless, I urge you not to turn off your thinking switches,

In the following example, I will illustrate how the three are connected: mind, thoughts, and focus. Consider the scenario where a camel driver is holding a camel with a rope, and a camel is walking behind him.

According to that illustration, the camel driver represents our focus, the rope represents our mind, and the camel represents our thought. To enter the flow state, we have to use this focus first. The mind produces thoughts related to this focus.

Let me give you an example. You want to write an article on rain. Therefore, we need to focus on this first. The mind produces thoughts related to the topic of rain.

I searched with a fascination for an example explaining the relationship between our mind and focus. I needed a simple illustration explaining the relationship between the mind and focus.

As your focus is on the topic of rain, your thoughts are related to

"

You're about to
discover an exciting
way to connect your
thoughts, mind and
focus. Its life
unlocking a vault of
endless possibilities.

DNA "

To enter the flow state......

To enter
the flow
state,
we have to
use this focus
first.
The mind
produces
thoughts
related to this
focus.

DNA

"

Are you looking to
broaden your
perspective and
strengthen your
relationship with
yourself?

"

DNA

the topic of rain. Those thoughts will start to enter your mind as you think. Your focus determines the direction of your thoughts. After a while, when you enter the flow state, the scenario changes, and you will be surprised. Before flow starts, the camel driver that is your focus was ahead of the camel that is your thoughts.

Once the flow starts ideas do not need to be led by a camel driver, that is your focus. Having done so, the camel, representing a group of arranged thoughts following the camel driver, has now moved forward, leaving behind the camel driver, the focus. The flow is a mental state where your focus follows your thoughts. Imagine a camel moving forward and a camel driver following the camel with a rope.

> **Now the situation has changed. As a result of the flow state, ideas do not need to be led by a camel driver that is focus.**

With a flow, there is no such thing as a difficult task. Get rid of the misperception that highly gifted people can only accomplish great pieces of work. Instead, we can attain our optimum performance with flow state concepts. While in the very present moment, while you are reading this book. Putting your hand on your heart is a way to feel it because I am saying it while putting it on my heart. I believe we are all gifted with the ability to acquire remarkable skills.

Many people believe that some people have God-given gifts of talents, and they are the only ones capable of doing things like that, I call that a disbelief. The idea of this book is to make you believe you are gifted with extraordinary mental skills.

There is no such thing as a
different task......

With a flow, there
is no such thing as
a difficult task.
Get rid of the
misperception that
highly gifted
people can only
accomplish great
pieces of work.
Instead, we can
attain our optimum
performance with
flow state
concepts.

DNA

Step 15

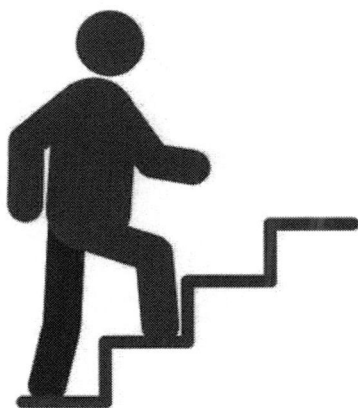

Why do we experience intense power in the flow state? How does it allow us to reach peak performance?

In next few pages
you're about to find out!

- Nature's golden law and secret: energy flows in directions where there is flow. What can you do to enhance your intelligence by using this law?

- The rapture of our minds is like a leaf on the waves of a river. Why do we need it?

- Is it possible to create the most powerful waves of our mind just as easily as they are in the ocean?

- A small fish in the Atlantic Ocean can withstand waves nine feet high

with the power it generates. How
can we provide that kind of power?

osmic secrets! Where there is a flow there is energy. Well, this is a very interesting aspect of a flow state, and we will now see it in the context of physical laws. Physics states that the direction of energy occurs in the direction of flow. This law applies to our mind flow as well. In the flow state an energy that arises in your mind just not remain limited to you. This energy creates a zone that does create a hidden deep spark within you. Its waves spread out from your being and from your mind into your whole surroundings.

If you are writing on paper, your paper and your pen become energised. The door and wall of your room, your chair, your table, the lamp on your table all become uplifted. You, the present time, and a place where you are will form a loop of intertwined energy. This network is super powerful.

You must have seen there are some fishes that can swim on the surface of the ocean and there are some fishes that can go to the depths of the ocean, so is the human flow state. This mental flow also has its depths and speed

Where there is a flow there is energy. Well, this is a very interesting aspect of a flow state, and we will now see it in the context of physical laws.

In the flow state......

In the flow state
an energy that
arises in your
mind just not
remain limited to
you. This energy
creates a zone
that does create
a hidden deep
spark within you

DNA

"

Nature's golden law
and secret: energy
flows in directions
where there is flow.
What can you do to
enhance your
intelligence by using
this law?

"

DNA

.Just like the flow of ocean waves has a direction, a speed, a height, and a depth. In the same way, mind flow state waves have a speed, height, and a depth, within this zone you will be able to dive far into the depths of your own mind. Even in deep waters you will be able to get far. But it takes practice. You must put a dedicated well-planned effort for it. Let me say here that research says that the deeper you go, the more unique and different your thoughts and ideas become.

At this point, I want to tell you a strong and powerful story. This is the story of a determined and focused heart, a small but a super strong heart. And it is the heart in the chest of a fish, the strength of that heart and mind is to be in a flow state. To know all about it, let's have a look at an epic life journey.

It is born in brackish waters and travels sometime after its birth to fresh waters. Into the deep seas. With passage of time, it has come hundreds and thousands of miles away in Atlantic Ocean.

There are some fishes that can swim on the surface of the ocean and there are some fishes that can go to the depths of the ocean, so the human flow state which is the thinking flow state. It is a state of mental flow, it also has depth and speed.

When the time comes for her to lay her eggs, then she makes a very interesting and surprising decision, that decision is to start a journey travelling back to her birthplace to lay eggs. But there is a big challenge. She is far away from where she was born. It is in her heart that she decides that she

"

Is it possible to create the most powerful waves of our mind just as easily as they are in the ocean?

"

DNA

will fight against the distance of thousands of miles across the deep waters and mighty waves of ocean and will return to her place of birth. To give birth to her children in the same place where she herself was born. And this is not just a fictional story this is a real-life story.

Now she embarks on a journey of thousands of miles. The first obstacle to overcome. the waves in the Atlantic Ocean. Waves are so high and powerful that they sometimes go as high as three to six meters. These waves are physically flowing against the direction of this fish's ultimate destination and goal. But the small yet strong and energetic heart of this fish is ready to fight these strongest waves flowing in the opposite direction.

You may have also noticed that some fish are fast swimmers and some are slow swimmers. We too can increase the speed and depth of our superpower flow after Learning our mental flow states.

The second surprising thing in this journey is to find out the direction of destination. She has come thousands of miles away from her birthplace, now for our mind to ponder how. a miracle happens, this fish finds its direction to its destination thousands of miles away. The possible science behind it. It is suggested that they have some electromagnetic receptors in their brain. These small devices help them to navigate. It is also said that every part of the earth has a secret electromagnetic signature. That is, every inch of the earth is sealed with an electric magnetic field. And it travels back to its birthplace using those seals as landmarks. Eventually with determined flow this fish gets to its destination and achieves the ultimate goal.

See the mircale......

See the miracle
that this fish
finds its
destination
thousands of
miles away. The
science behind it.
It is said about
him that he may
have some such
electromagnetic
receptors in his
brain.

DNA

Step 16

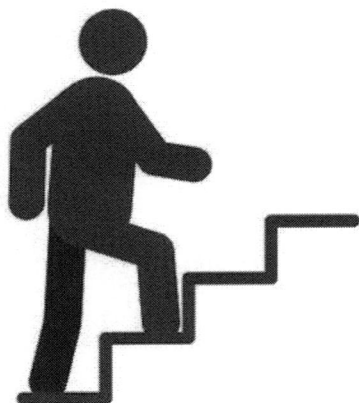

Walk like Darwin-
to think Like Darwin
How walks get you
in Zone- and can
make you super
intelligent

In next few pages you're about to find out!

- There comes a point when you start reading your hidden mind while you are walking; why do you reach that point in your walking?

- The switch of ideas is turned on by walking. But how?

- A look at how walking transformed Charles Dickens and William Wordsworth and other geniuses.

- During walking, what precious neurochemicals and growth factors are released?

- **Research reveals how walking affects the size of people's brains even over age 60.**

It is inevitable that there will come a time when you begin to have a fast-moving mind as you walk. Then while you are walking, there's a moment when you begin to read your hidden mind. It's like listening to your inner voice, and suddenly you become aware of all your thoughts and feelings. You start to make connections between different ideas and come up with creative solutions. This can be a powerful tool for self-exploration and growth.

This is the moment when you start coming up with incredibly original thoughts in solitude. It could be argued that those long walks that lead to Flow essentially turn the creative switch into what we could call an idea's switch.

Charles Dickens was a writer, social commentator, and walker. Following his writing for the day, from 9 a.m. until 2 p.m., he would walk for 20 or 30 miles. Dickens strolled London streets until morning when he couldn't sleep at night. The friends of Dickens used to get upset when he walked so much. They guessed that he had a passion for hiking. But frankly, walking did a lot for him.

Dickens wrote more than a dozen large and well-known novels, several collections of short stories, a few plays, and even some non-fiction books. According to the man himself, if he does not walk "far and fast." Then he will "burst and perish" with the psychological burden of silence. Without walking, he would probably go crazy.

It is inevitable that there will come a time when you begin to have a fast-moving mind as you walk. Then while you are walking, there's a moment when you begin to read your mind

Charles Dickens was a......

Charles Dickens
was a writer,
social
commentator,
and walker.
Following his
writing for the
day, from
9 a.m.
until 2 p.m.,
he would walk
for 20 or 30
minutes.

DNA

"

There comes a point
when you start
reading your hidden
mind while you are
walking; why do you
reach that point in
your walking?

"

DNA

Walking helps you remove the dust from your mind. Researchers have shown that animals that run on a treadmill for a long time create new connections between their brain cells. There is also a significant increase in its size when it comes to walkers. It seems to work like a high-speed processor.

The poet William Wordsworth travelled nearly 175,000 miles throughout his life and maintained a brilliant writing career. Wordsworth's walk was as if he were following in his footsteps. The process of walking was "indivisible" from writing poetry. Both were rhythmic meters required in both. He needed to walk to write.

Walking was a lifelong exercise for Darwin. As a young man in 1826, Darwin set out on a North Wales trek with friends, walking about thirty miles a day with bags on his back. In his autobiography, he noted. Even as a child, he was known for his long walks. The taste of loneliness drove him to walk, he wrote. On one afternoon, as he was returning from an excursion to the old castles of Shrewsbury, he fell seven or eight feet. The path was over. He wrote, 'I was often quite absorbed, yet Darwin walked every day in the sun or the pouring rain at the age of sixty.'

> The poet William Wordsworth travelled nearly 175,000 miles throughout his life and maintained a brilliant writing career. Wordsworth's walk was as if he were following in his footsteps.

As a neurologist, I want to tell you about a grey substance in your brain. We call this grey matter. Additionally, there is white-looking tissue. Typically, the brain's white matter is made up of a network of fibres that connect the different cells in the brain together.

Here is a straightforward example that I would like to share with you. The grey matter of our brain is like a computer. White matter

"

The switch of ideas
is turned on by
walking. But how?

"

DNA

is the cables that connect everything and transmit signals from one place to another.

Now that we know this, I would like to tell you about research done on 250 seniors over the age of 60 who were tested for cognitive fitness. To determine their mental and intellectual abilities, MRI brain scans were conducted on each of them. Then they looked at their grey matter and their white matter. Through this research, team discovered the

fantastic result that grey matter size increased in the elderly who walked daily for six months. This indicates that walking is an effective way to improve cognitive functioning, even for elderly people. The research team also found that walking improved the elderly's reaction time and attention span. And as a result, their mental and intellectual abilities improved. The group of elders who walked had a better memory than those who did not.

Now that we know this, I would like to tell you about research done on 250 seniors over the age of 60 who were tested for neurotic fitness. To determine their mental and intellectual abilities, MRI brain scans were conducted on each of them. Then they took a look at their grey matter and their white matter

Let me now share with you another incredible thing that I believe will be able to help you change the course of your life forever. There is now evidence that certain precious chemicals are also produced when we walk, and scientists have confirmed this. Some of these factors are called neurotrophic factors, and one contains a valuable chemical known as BDNF, Brain-Derived Neurotrophic Factor, which is a type of a growth factor for our brains.

The chemical can be considered a molecular fertiliser for the brain. When fertilisers are added to fields and orchards, they greatly enhance the crops grown in the areas. They make them healthier and multiply the harvest in many ways. In the same way, these brain fertilisers fertilise the crops of our thoughts and the soil of our brains. They contribute to creating neuronal networks. By stimulating the growth of neurons and synapses, they increase our cognitive functioning, enabling us to think, reason, and remember better. Additionally, they help to reduce the effects of ageing on the brain, making it possible for us to stay sharp and alert even in old age.

When such neural networks are formed, our brain's processor works as fast as a computer's processor. This helps us to think quickly and solve problems. It also helps us to make better decisions and learn new skills. The more neurons we can create, the more powerful our brain becomes.

Let me now share......

Let me now
share with you
another incredible
thing that I believe
will be able to help
you change the
course of your life
forever. There is now
evidence that
certain precious
chemicals are also
produced when we
walk, and scientists
have confirmed this.

DNA

Step 17

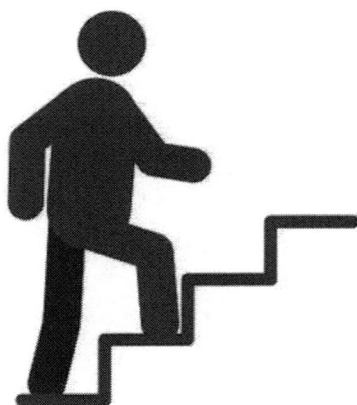

A hidden power of Mother Earth's electromagnetic energy that can influence our minds must be revealed

In next few pages
you're about to find out!

- No one has ever told you about the power of the Earth that you can use for your mind and thinking.

- Your current location influences how you think.

- How does it affect your thinking and mind? Electromagnetic energy can be found on Earth's surface in what ways?

- Introducing Showman Resonance, an amazing scientific secret. In what ways can electromagnetic waves

around the Earth affect our
brains? Amazing research?

- Get in touch with Mother Earth
again, but why?

You are about to find out something extraordinary. It has never been mentioned to you before. However, it is this very fact that will change the way and where you choose to be in life.

The place where you are physically located has a significant impact on you. This could have a substantial effect on the way you think. Please let me explain more about what I mean by this statement.

There is a wave of electromagnetic energy circling the planet. Magnetic waves are a part of the electromagnetic field. There are electrons in our Earth's atmosphere that can form magnetic waves. These are the waves which are responsible for the electromagnetic network. The frequencies of electromagnetic waves are about similar to some of brain waves.

I strongly believe our brainwaves are affected by these electromagnetic waves, just as ocean waves are affected by lunar electromagnetic and gravitational waves. In the lower ionosphere of Earth, there is a set of frequencies called the Schumann resonance produced by electromagnetic waves.

Lightning and thunderstorms create frequencies between 7.83 Hz and 33.8 Hz, known as the Earth's heartbeat ". The Schumann Resonance has been studied for its effect on the human mind. Laurentian University researchers published a 2016 paper that found that 238 measurements over 3.5 years from 184

Our brainwaves are affected by these electromagnetic waves, just as ocean waves are affected by these Lunar electromagnetic and gravitational waves.

"

No one has ever told
you about the power
of the Earth that you
can use for your mind
and thinking

"

DNA.

individuals showed some surprising similarities in electromagnetic field strength and spectral patterns generated by the human brain and earth-ionospheric cavity.

Schumann's Resonance is believed to act as a bridge between the conscious and the subconscious mind. It is thought that the Earth network's waves can affect the brain waves for deep focus and attention. This network can enable us to tap into our subconscious mind and access extrasensory perceptions.

> **Surprising** similarities **in** electromagnetic field **strength** and **spectral patterns** generated **by** the **human** brain and earth-**ionospheric acavity**

Please get in the process of connecting it to your brain waves. By associating our brain waves with electromagnetic waves of Mother Earth, we can help our brain waves change for better ideas. Find a place in nature to connect to the subtle and faint yet powerful EM waves.

Let me tell you something you may find very interesting ; several animals exhibit magnetoreception, i.e., the ability to detect electromagnetic waves, including pigeons, dogs, trout, bees, turtles, and salamanders. Researchers have been trying to find out if humans have similar powers for decades.

Earth affects thinking; let me explain how? Using a technology known as transcranial magnetic stimulation (TMS) makes it possible to therapeutically alter the activity of specific brain waves in a targeted area of the brain by creating a magnetic field. We must wonder how the Earth's natural electromagnetic field influences our thinking and emotions in light of the effects on cognitive processes.

Could a change in this field affect opinions and moods on a global scale? Is it possible to alter our brain electromagnetic fields? More

"

Introducing Showman
Resonance, an
amazing scientific
secret. In what ways
can electromagnetic
waves around the
Earth affect our
brains?
"

DNA

Please get in the process......

Please get in the
process of connecting
it to your brain
waves. By associating
our brain
waves with
electromagnetic
waves, we can
help our brain waves
change
for better ideas Find
a place in nature to
connect to the
EM waves

DNA

answers to these questions will be revealed in time. I know, deep down, that Mother Earth is an electromagnetic being, just as we all are. Our brains and bodies have a particular type of iron that can detect these EM waves. I believe when we connect with nature, our energetic frequency oscillates at the same frequency as the Earth's vibration, which is unsurprising.

> Our **brains** and bodies have a **particular** type of iron that can potentially detect **these** EM waves. When we **connect** with nature, our energetic **frequency oscillates** at the same **frequency** as the **Earth's** vibration, which is unsurprising.

Connecting with mother nature and the Earth brings us to life. Therefore, it breathes life into our lives. Additionally, it cleanses and rejuvenates our energy field. Mother Earth's frequency is one of the most potent healing frequencies on the planet. It is perfectly configured for human beingness to be at their best. Undoubtedly, the Earth is like an enormous battery - when we connect with it, we are recharged!

Take time to connect with the Earth through a grounding meditation. I am happy to share a straightforward grounding method, no matter where you are. Find a spot connected to the Earth, such as walking with your feet on grass, soil, or on a beach. Just have a deep sense of connection with the Earth through your feet. The roots of your being sink into the ground and connect with the Earth.

The moment you feel connected, you will feel the pure energy of lovely Earth rising through you. Your body will be infused with earthly powers if you allow her energy to flow through your base. There is a belief that physical contact between our bodies and the Earth is essential for our health and well-being. The concept is called "earthing" or "grounding" and is based on the belief that the Earth's surface contains free electrons that can be transferred to the human body by direct contact. As a result, these electrons act as antioxidants that help neutralise free radicals in our bodies and prevent inflammation.

There is a belief......

There is a
belief that
physical
contact
between
our bodies
and
the Earth is
essential for
our health
and
well-being

DNA

Step 18

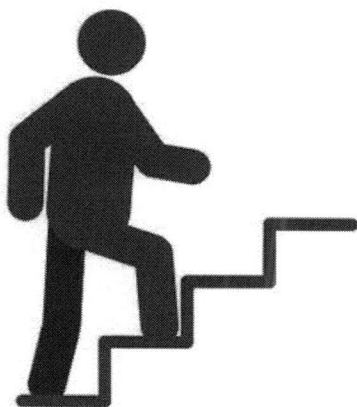

Getting the best out of our brain during the Divine Hours of the Night- How it works?

In next few pages you're about to find out!

- Do the hours between three and five in the night have any unusual powers? During this period, why you can experience a heightened awareness of the energy around you.

- Which makes this time of night powerful? This time is known as the 'Divine Hour'. It is the time when the veil between the physical and spiritual worlds is thinnest.

- How did my father, Sehba Akhtar, use this hour of the night for poetry? He would sit atop a creative hill and write, letting the

Divine Hour energy flow through him and onto the paper.

- What is the point of spending one night a week alone with a pen and paper? to tap into innermost thoughts and feelings.

- Why did such a genius like Picasso and a brilliant poet like Ghalib use the night for artistic work? Why night brings out the highest taste in creative minds.

The early hours before dawn are special and divine hours filled with energy waves coming to our planet from beyond. It has yet to be discovered. Because of these energy waves, we will likely have "peak moments" in our thinking lives. There will be times when we can reach a peak state much more quickly than at any other time throughout the day.

My study of the lives of the world's significant achievers and icons of self-actualisation has led me to the conclusion that the early morning hours, the twilight zone between night and day, are the most energised times of the day, a period when a deep connection with one's innermost self-most likely to happen.

These divine hours are as powerful as a black hole in the cosmos. Imagine what could happen to you if the force of a black hole possessed you. Every aspect of your life would be drawn towards it. Nothing could escape. Or detach from it. Consequently, each step you take would have a seamless flow towards your goals, making you feel self-confident in what you're doing.

As you gain more peak experiences, you will become more transformed. To find and serve our higher purpose, we need to spend time surrounding ourselves with ourselves. To start your day with a bang, you must connect with yourself first thing in the morning. This will enable you to be in your most inspired and powerful state. It would be best if you reconnected with your purpose.

> *The early morning hours are special and divine hours filled with energy waves coming to our planet from beyond. It has yet to be discovered.*

These divine hours are ......

These divine
hours are as
powerful as
a black hole
in the
cosmos.
Imagine what
could happen
to you if the
force of a
black hole
possessed
you.

DNA

"

Do the hours between three and five in the night have any power? Could it be due to the electromagnetic field network? During this period, you can experience a heightened awareness of the energy around you.

"

DNA

Why do darkness and silence affect our minds' creativity and productivity? The waves that run on the surface of our brains become more robust simultaneously. Let's take a closer look at this concept.

There is no doubt that the darkness of night and its vibes have the power and ability to alter our brain waves. I know this from experience. Many of you will have a similar experience when preparing for exams, understanding something, and memorising a subject in school and college. It is most effective to study at night.

> **There is no doubt that the darkness of night and its vibes have the power and ability to alter our brain waves. I know this from experience**

Getting up earlier on those nights also gives us more time. The night's romance enriches our minds and souls in many ways. A study has been conducted by the University of Milan in Italy. There were young students involved in the study. Students who studied at night performed better on the tests than their average peers.

When Robin Sharma wrote his book 5 am Club, people worldwide began to realise the importance of 5 am. This led to a revolution that changed people's lives. From Obama to Steve Jobs, many people used to start their day at 4 am. This early start to the day was made popular by influential figures and is a great way to get a head start on the day. Often referred to as conscious or inspirational hours, these hours occur between 3 am and 5 am and are believed to be mindful and inspiring for many reasons. Hence, they are also known as divine hours.

Explaining this secret rule is challenging, but my intuitive estimation leads me to believe it. Let me explain. There is an electromagnetic network, which consists of electric and magnetic waves around

"

Do the hours between three and five in the night have any power? Could it be due to the electromagnetic field network? During this period, you can experience a heightened awareness of the energy around you.

"

DNA

our mother earth. As a result of the network, brain waves' speed and rhythm are altered so that many extrasensory abilities are unlocked. They can detect extrasensory perceptions.

Explaining this secret rule is challenging, but my intuitive estimation leads me to believe it. Let me explain

Ghalib is the Einstein of human emotions and the most celebrated Urdu poet of all time. By giving the language multi literary colours, and various unique angles, he immortalised Urdu. He used to have poetic arrival at night time. To memorise these poems, he tied multiple knots on the corner of his shirt, which allowed him to recall them in the morning.

I have also witnessed the poetic arrival. In the middle of the night, I remember my father, Sehba Akhtar Sahib, sitting on a chair, smoking a cigarette, holding a pen and paper, and writing in a trance-like state. The best poems he wrote were written at night when he woke up. A large part of Naatia Kalam Iqra and the Naats were composed during these inspired night moments.

Whether you are a poet or not, you can still live a revolutionary life by bringing powerful brain waves with different approaches. Ideas and inspiration are necessary if you want a change in your life.

To achieve your goals, think outside the box. One way to do that is to dedicate these periods to yourself during the solitude of magical night time. The practice should be repeated at least once a week, preferably twice a week. Your efforts will be rewarded. It will prove to you what I mean when you start doing it. It would be best to have a pen and a topic to reflect on.

You can form a connection with yourself, your paper, and your pen during the energising and engrossing hours of the night. You will witness this connection, and the creative ideas will flow on paper.

In his lifetime, Pablo Picasso produced nearly 16,000 paintings and drawings - an incredible amount, made possible by his late-night work habits. When he was young, he spent all night painting while his poet roommate slept. Eventually, Picasso moved to a studio in Montparnasse as his popularity grew. However, his routine has remained unchanged.

I firmly believe that the electromagnetic spectrum around this planet during night time enhances the powerful waves in your brain. At night, the electromagnetic spectrum allows for a surge of creativity and imagination, unlocking our minds and allowing us to explore new and exciting ideas. The late night and early morning hours are divine. These brain waves have a great deal of power use them. Make the most of these hours to manifest your desires and create the life you want.

> To achieve your goals, think outside the box. One way to do that is to dedicate these periods to yourself during the nighttime.

At night the electromagnetic
spectrum allows ......

At night, the
electromagnetic
spectrum allows
for a surge of
creativity and
imagination,
unlocking our
minds and
allowing us to
explore new and
exciting ideas

DNA

Step 19

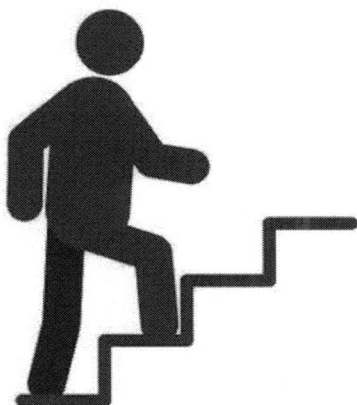

Getting great ideas, one of the best times of the day What is happening in our brain just before we completely wake up?

In next few pages you're about to find out!

- Since birth till now the most precious time of your day is easily wasted by you.

- Why did Edison and Tesla will hold an iron ball before going to sleep?

- How should one use the powerful waves of the mind immediately after waking up?

We mainly don't allow our minds to flash ideas and capture them. A special time zone passes over minds twice daily for a brief period. Without our knowledge, these precious time zones are drained without remorse.

I want to elaborate on the time spell I am talking about; this is the time just after waking up. It is the moment when our brains begin to switch from sleep to wakefulness.

At the borders of our awareness lies a twilight zone. The junction between sleep and awakening is called the hypnopompic stage. In this state of altered consciousness, we can access ideas and insights that may remain hidden in our waking state.

This is a powerful time zone to explore our inner world and uncover our creativity. It can also be a valuable tool for problem-solving, as our dreams can provide us with alternative perspectives and solutions.

Our brains are very powerful in this time zone because alpha waves flood our brains just before completely waking up. Once fully awakened, more ordinary waves capture and control our brains.
These fast waves are for day-to-day decision- making and everyday thoughts but not for the best ideas. It is a brief but excellent opportunity that we all have every day. It is so helpful that many have used it to change their world and the world outside them. They used this period as creative duration.

> **In this state of altered consciousness, we can access ideas and insights that may remain hidden in our waking state**

Our brains are very powerful ......

Our brains are
very powerful in
this time zone
because
alpha waves flood
our brains just
before
waking up.
Once fully
awakened, more
ordinary waves
capture and
control our
brains.

DNA

"

Why did Edison and
Tesla etc. sleep
holding an iron
ball before going
to sleep?
"

DNA

This supercharged creative period has been used by geniuses like Newton, Edison and Tesla. It has been written that most of them used to grab an iron ball before slipping off to sleep. This was so that as soon as they fell asleep, the ball would fall from their hands and wake them up, and they would be in this zone. This was to help them enter a altered state of alertness and focus. This would enable their creative brain waves to flow, giving them the ability to do the incredible works of genius they are remembered for today.

During this zone, they will let their minds get out-of-the-box ideas. At this point, at this twilight phase of our conciseness. Our frontal lobe is quiet and not fully awake and our connection with space and time is not established.

I'll share my hypothesis with you so that you can gain a deeper understanding of it. Certain areas in the brain are full of intelligence and are typically kept silent due to the rule of the frontal lobe. The secret is that these areas of the brain, if accessed and stimulated correctly can unlock powerful insights and ideas. This is not available when relying solely on the frontal lobe and prison of logic.

> **As person transits from a state of sleep to a state of awakening, the sense of "here" and now" changes from the real world to the world of dreams.**

The twilight zone allows them to express their views freely. This is because your frontal lobe is still asleep. However, you're partially awake, along with a few suppressed areas of the brain that are normally quietened by the dictatorial rule of the frontal lobe.

As person transits from a state of sleep to a state of awakening, the sense of "here" and now" changes from the real world to the world of Ideas. This is due to the presence of unique alpha waves. When

"

How should one use the powerful waves of the mind immediately after waking up?

"

DNA

this happens, complex questions can be answered by generating many ideas.

Be sure to think about the subject before going to sleep. Sleep on the problem or question you want to answer, and then think about it in the same twilight zone the following day. You will be surprised to find answers to your questions using this junction.

In addition, this time can also be used to do self-hypnosis to eliminate imperfections from your mind, if you wish. In this robust junction, you can highlight your abilities because, at this time, the centre of your ego is not dictating. There is a greater chance of finding yourself when the centre of fear is asleep. In addition to taking your advice, your higher self is also ready to do so.

Sleep on the problem ......

Sleep on the
problem or
question you
want to answer,
and then think
about it in the
same twilight
zone the
following day.
You will be
surprised to find
answers to your
questions
using this
junction.

DNA

Step 20

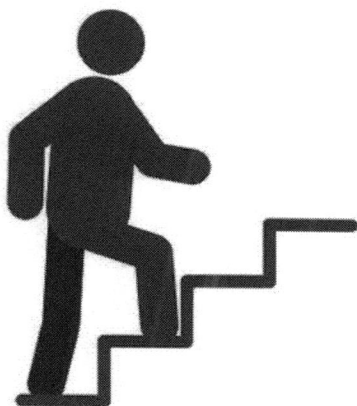

Thinking with closed eyes: why does it work for geniuses and how will it work for you?

In next few pages
you're about to find out!

- Have you seen the pictures of Einstein and Alama Iqbal thinking while closed-eyed?

- Do geniuses and thinkers often think with their eyes closed?

- When recalling a memory, why do people close their eyes?

- The secret reveals what happens to our brain waves when we close our eyes and think!

When I was growing up, I saw pictures of famous thinkers who often closed their eyes while they were still wide awake and thinking.

You must have seen during his later years, Allama Iqbal is often seen sitting on a chair and resting his head on the other hand while he thinks with his eyes closed. In this way, we have images of Einstein thinking with his eyes closed when he was a young man; we can examine these images on search engines.

I wanted to know why these great thinkers do that. Recently, I discovered an answer to this intriguing question. My research discovered that great thinkers, creators, poets, and scientists often close their eyes during their working hours, consciously or unconsciously. Artistry, ingenuity, and creativity could significantly increase due to eye-closed thinking in everyday life. How it happens, let's dig into it.

There are a few basic and simple things that you need to understand about brain functioning to be able to grasp this simple secret.

Undoubtedly, our eyes are one of the most vital sources of establishing a connection to the external world.

> I wanted to know why these great thinkers do that. Recently, I discovered an answer to this intriguing question.

However, when our eyes are closed while we are awake, the link to our inner world of creativity and intelligence can be established. Opening our inner eye. By allowing ourselves to open our inner eyes, we can tap into a realm of wisdom and understanding of what is hidden.

242

"

Have you seen the
pictures of Einstein
and Alama Iqbal
thinking while closed-
eyed?

"

DNA

There are a few basic ......

There are
a few basic
and simple
things that you
need to
understand
about brain
functioning to
be
able to
grasp this
simple
secret

DNA

"
The secret reveals what happens to our brain waves when we close our eyes and think!

"
DNA

It has been observed that some individuals often close their eyes when recalling an old memory or an event. Our inner journey will take us into what is hidden inside the brain and reach some areas we cannot usually access.

Significant electrochemical changes happen in our brains and minds when we close our eyes. To understand this further, let me tell you that when we wake up in the morning, the surface of our brains is filled with high-speed brain waves, which are running at high speeds continuously. Known as beta waves, these high-speed brain waves are essential for our day-to-day problem-solving, but they do not let us come up with big ideas and unique solutions in their presence.

When our eyes are closed while we are awake, the link to our inner world of creativity and intelligence can be established

After we close our eyes, the alpha waves develop, occupy our brain surface and operate our brains. With the help of these waves, the areas of the brain that were locked down by beta waves are reached and accessible. It is these brain waves that break the lockdown on the brain.

During the past few years, considerable research has been conducted on creativity and intelligence in general. An interesting study examined the phenomenon of coming up with ideas while one's eyes are closed. Is it able to influence the thinking process in any significant way?

As part of their research, the researchers divided the participants into eyes open thinking group and a blindfolded-thinking group, the participants from both groups were asked to come up with a new name for some business products. Research results group who thought while eyes closed much better in branding names.

"

Have you seen the pictures of Einstein and Alama Iqbal thinking while closed-eyed?

"

DNA

If you would like to perform better, you can use the technique during work and routine and think for a few minutes with your eyes closed, only for a few moments. To create a revolution of alpha waves in your brain, close your eyes while you focus your mind.

If you would Like......

If you would
Like to perform
better, you can use
the technique during
work and routine and
think for a
few minutes
with your
eyes closed,
only for a few
moments. To create
a revolution of
alpha waves in your
brain, close your
eyes while you focus
your mind

DNA

Step 21

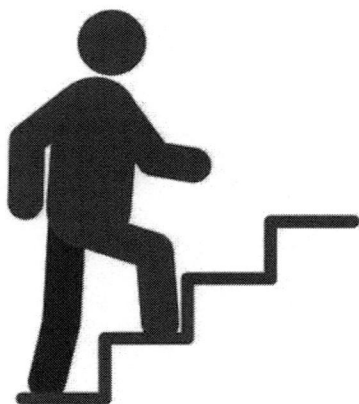

Discover the wonders of daydreaming - Visualise your daydreams every day, but why?

In next few pages
you're about to find out!

- Despite being wide awake, you should start dreaming, but why? Based on my research on daydreaming!

- A novel concept I have developed is called "Daydream meditation."

- How did Einstein's daydreams change our world forever? He famously visualised himself riding on a beam of light, which led him to develop?

- Are you interested in finding out how to access the most intelligent parts of your brain?

- **Try closing your eyes and dreaming of success, but why?**

Is daydreaming good for you? Yes, it is; in Neuroscience, one of the unique ways to access your creativity. When researchers explored the characteristics of creative minds and questioned whether daydreaming could enhance your ability to be creative and intelligent, yes, that's right.

Creativity certainly increases. The basis of my claim is that when we dream, different parts of our brains become active, and accessing information beyond our restricted logical reach is possible. This creative insight often leads to solutions to problems you didn't even consider.

Einstein is a big name in daydreaming. One of the secrets is that a few hours after Einstein's death, Thomas Harvey, the pathologist who performed the autopsy, removed Einstein's brain without his family's permission and against Einstein's wishes. After hiding them for many years, he finally sent parts of the brain to other scientists to study and unravel the mystery of Einstein's intellectual abilities.

Studies have shown that Einstein's brain, compared to other brains, has a higher proportion of glial cells in one part of the association cortex, which is responsible for combining and rearranging information from multiple parts of the brain. This was probably the result of Einstein spending so much time looking at and solving complex scientific problems creatively, ultra-logically designing and editing his daydreams to answer the universe's most complicated questions.

> Creativity certainly increases. The basis of my claim is that when we dream. As different parts of our brains become active

"

Are you interested in finding out how to access the most intelligent parts of your brain? Are you curious about unlocking your hidden potential?

"

DNA

Studies have shown that......

Studies have
shown that
Einstein's brain,
compared to
other brains, has
a higher
proportion of
glial cells in
one part of the
association
cortex, which is
responsible for
combining

DNA

Einstein also dreamed during the day. At the age of 15, he dropped out of school. Einstein dropped out of school because his teachers disapproved of the visual thinking process of visual Imagination for learning. These skills became the basis of his thinking. Einstein said, "Imagination is more important than knowledge." It is no coincidence that Einstein began to use thought experiments around this time, which changed his thoughts about his future experiences.

In one of these waking dreams while he was sitting on a bench in the city. The idea came, and he started daydreaming based on this idea. He was looking at the tower clock and the hands of the clock moving. He began to dream that he was riding a bicycle and riding fast in the opposite direction at a very high speed that exceeded the speed of light.

> **Ultra-Logically designing and editing his day dreams to answer the universe's most complicated questions.**
> **I do not doubt that Einstein also dreamed during the day**

Then the wave of light coming toward his eyes after hitting the hands of the clock will not be able to reach his eyes because the speed of his bicycle has exceeded the speed of light. He will see the hands of the clock stand still in one place. Based on this and based on such day-to-day dreams, Einstein solved many great mysteries.

Albert Einstein used to say: whether they are written or spoken, words or language do not play a role in my thinking system. According to Albert Einstein, thinking experiments are done in the Imagination. We set some situations, observe what happens, and try to draw the correct conclusion. In this way, intellectual experiences resemble real experiences, except they are brain experiences.

"

Try closing your
eyes and dreaming
of success, but why?
We can use them to
push us to strive for
our goals and take
the first steps
toward achieving
our ambitions

"

DNA

Let me tell you this, all the fundamental wise ideas have already been thought of thousands of times. But to truly make them our own, we must re-think them honestly until they take root in our intellect.

A recent study by the Georgia Institute of Technology supports Kaufmann and Gregor's that people who report daydreaming often have higher intellectual and creative abilities scores. - In fact, their brains were more efficient. According to another study, researchers at the University of Southern California have identified brain areas where humans acquire meaning. It was discovered that we seek meaning by interpreting life stories and experiences.

> A recent study by the Georgia Institute of Technology supports Kaufmann and Gregor's that people who report day dreaming often have higher - In fact, their brains were more efficient

We only see a small part of reality with our limited senses and consciousness. In addition, there is a constant flow of energy throughout the universe. There are no simple words or ideas that can capture the complexity and flow of this movement. The only way to become enlightened is to allow flow of its meaning and purpose.

Many studies have shown that daydreaming can reduce stress and anxiety, improve problem-solving skills, enhance creativity, and reduce stress and anxiety. Setting and achieving goals are also improved by taking time to think for pleasure. It may seem counterintuitive, but studies continue to indicate that letting your mind wander in directed daydreaming may be just what you need to move forward.

While your mind is directed towards a goal directed and answer seeking daydreaming, you use a variety of brain functions. Two networks work simultaneously in your brain: the executive problem-solving and involuntary sunbconcoius creativity networks. By activating these brain areas, we can gain access to information that was previously unavailable or dormant.

I encourage you to construct a daydream to find solutions by using your brain's para-logical super-intelligent centres. If you dream, you are not imprisoned or confined within the box, regardless of whether you are dreaming while awake or asleep. As a result of these flow-state-driven daydreaming exercises, you can find many ways to achieve your goals and solve your challenges.

I encourage you to......

I encourage you
to construct a day
dream to find
solutions by using
your brain's
para-logical super-
intelligent centres.
If you dream, you
are not
imprisoned or
confined within the
box, regardless of
whether you are
dreaming while
awake or asleep

DNA

Step 22

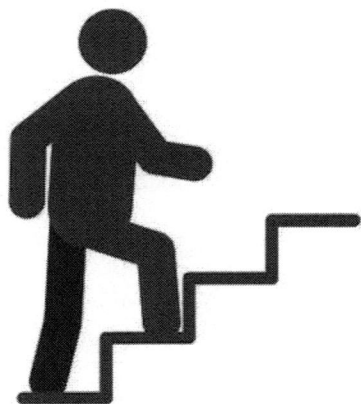

An innovative hypothesis for driving intelligence: connecting to the past, present, and future creative auras

In next few pages
you're about to find out!

- What is an aura or halo of power around us? And how is it created?

- How can the aura of energy around highly intelligent people and those who are at the pinnacle of their craft empower your mind?

- How can it benefit you to be in the company of such people?

- Can these geniuses and masters of their art send waves of wisdom to your brain on how this theory of mine can surprisingly benefit you?

- When thousands of millions of birds flying in the sky, without talking to each other, how do they go around in a circle with great speed?

As far as I am concerned, the aura can be described as a circle of energy surrounding us. Let me explain it is an undetectable energy that surrounds us and is produced by everyone differently. Some people can feel this energy, which I believe reveal the deeper aspects of an individual's mind and soul.

It is said that an individual's aura can change and evolve over time, depending on their experiences and the energy they absorb from the environment. This energy is subtle yet powerful and does convey messages to impact our existence and our environment.

I believe those who are masters of their fields and who have achieved excellence by working extremely hard over the years also develop an aura of strong energy around them.

It is very much possible that a form of energy field surrounds our brains that has yet to be identified by science. When people come into close contact with masters of purity and creativity, they may experience esoteric phenomena explained by this "field". I hypothesise that the electromagnetic field is difficult to detect due to the limited technology available today. These unique spiritual-physical vibes are transmitted to the people around. To me, it is a secret to be unravelled.

> I believe those who are **masters** of their fields and who have achieved excellence by working extremely hard over the years also develop an aura of strong energy around them.

A person's aura of energy can be an excellent motivator and help open more imaginative ideas and perspectives. It can help unlock

"

How can the aura of energy around highly intelligent people and those who are at the pinnacle of their craft empower your mind?

"

DNA

A person's aura of energy......

A person's aura of
energy can be an
excellent
motivator and
help open
up more
imaginative ideas
and perspectives.
It can help
unlock
creative potential
and find
innovative
solutions

DNA

creative potential and find innovative solutions.

How they're transmitted and how those around them perceive them is also something that remains a secret. Even if you cannot converse with someone, you could have hit a vibration of inspiration or motivation that hit you. That feeling of connection, even if unspoken, is something that transcends spoken language, distance, and time.

This is why many people feel connected even when they don't speak the same language. This connection is so powerful that it can actually be experienced across physical barriers. It can even be felt when people are miles apart due to the invisible bond of waves created between them. This is to illustrate how strong a bond is shared between people.

As I have, there is probably something that you have noticed about flocks of birds flying across the sky. Hundreds of them can change directions in a fraction of a second without any explicit communication

A person with this type of super-brain can directly transmit vibes of deeper wisdom to another individual within their company. In My view, this can be achieved by the mechanism known as direct Brain-to-Brain communication, which is possible to achieve.

Let me explain what brain-to-brain communication is and how it works. According to the hypothesis, it is a form of direct communication between animals without using the usual sensory channels through which messages can be conveyed. I have an example to explain it further. As I have, there is probably something that you have noticed about flocks of birds flying across the sky. Hundreds and thousands of them can change directions in a

"

When thousands of
millions of birds flying
in the sky, without
talking to each other,
how do they go around in
a circle with great
speed? Amazing
revelation.

"

DNA

fraction of a second without any explicit communication. It is possible only if there is some communication, likely electromagnetic waves transmitted between birds. At super-fast speeds, hundreds and thousands of birds are changing directions seamlessly.

A few scientific studies have shown that different animals can communicate directly through their brains. The possibility of direct brain-to-brain communication (DBBC) between animals and humans has been reported recently, which goes beyond the conventional five senses.

There is an excellent example of the validity of DBBC demonstrated by recording similar patterns of action potentials in the brain cortex of two animals

There is an excellent example of the validity of DBBC demonstrated by recording similar patterns of action potentials in the brain cortex of two animals. Action potentials are electrical activities that occur in the brain's cells. The magnetic field that results from the action potentials created in brain cells is one of the mechanisms by which one animal's brain can affect another's brain. Cryptochrome, a chemical pigment found in the retina and different brain areas, has been shown to sense magnetic fields and convert them into action potentials.

Scientists believe that brain cell iron particles can act as magnetic field receptors. These unusual iron particles could potentially sense the brain's feeble magnetic field. According to a study published recently, there is a possibility that the feeble magnetic field within the brain of an animal can transmit vital and accurate information to that of another animal's brain.

Since animals can communicate directly with their brains, why can't humans? This raises the question of why humans must rely on verbal or written communication to convey their thoughts and feelings when animals can communicate without a language. I would like to introduce you to another paradigm I have been contemplating for a while.

The aura is energy, and energy cannot be destroyed, but it can take on different forms. If there is a strong desire, it is still possible to connect with the minds of geniuses who may not be physically present in this world. However, their mental energies have been preserved in this universe as an aura. To this end, we can use this aura to channel the knowledge of past geniuses and tap into their wisdom.

The Aura is energy......

The Aura is
energy, and
energy cannot be
destroyed, but it
can take on
different forms.
If there is a
strong desire, it
is still possible
to connect with
the minds of
geniuses who
may not be
physically
present
in this world

DNA

Step 23

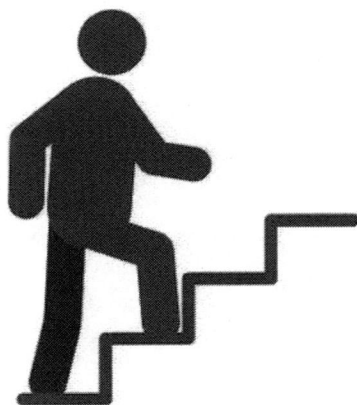

Master the mind's mastering flow by unraveling mystical mental codes

In next few pages you're about to find out!

- Where is the key to your mental treasures?

- How can words and phrases magically become keys to the locked treasures of the mind?

- If we must open the closed doors of the mind and their locks, what flames must be awakened in our mind?

- And how will they melt the chains binding the mind, but how? Based on the research.

We can unlock our mind's hidden locks by searching for magical phrases, master memories, or even pictures from the present, past, or even a future. The following example will give you insight into what I mean by that. My father used to tell us, " May you achieve big in your life", as a slogan of a recognition of efforts whether trivial or immense . It was him we grew up listening to. Let me give you some context for how it has affected us throughout our lives.

 You must have seen the typical safety locks usually opened by a unique code. In the same way, a phrase can act as a code to unlock any mind potential that has been locked. Our responsibility is to search for a magical phrase that can unlock the potential of our minds.

The truth is that there are many codes in the form of phrases that can be interpreted as a mission statement about your life. Any of these can be used as a universal motivational prescription for resolving any mental challenges you encounter. Because there are different codes and keys to go with various locks, it is possible for a particular code that works for you may not work for me, and the same goes for what could work for me may not work for you.

It is simple; all you have to do is look for codes that touches your heart and soul.

> **We can unlock your mind's hidden locks by searching for magical phrases, memories, or even pictures from the present, past, or future**

Once you have found those unique magical phrases or codes, please continue to read, listen, and try to internalise what they mean. It might be possible that you have been given a unique

"

Where is the key to your mental treasures?

DNA **"**

message passed on to you, which will serve as an inspiration and insight.

You do not need to do anything other than use this flame to invoke the power of super consciousness and then repeat it day and day out throughout your life every day. This will become an endless perpetual source of super energy for you. If these phrases or collection of words were said to you by a person from present, past or future then there it would be even more benefit to this idea if you could hear these phrases in their voices in your mind.

If we want to unlock the potential of our minds, we need a spark of inner flame to melt the locks and unleash the potential within. After a flame with a super energy of this magnitude, your brain will be opened up to new pathways and opportunities for uplifting trajectories. With the use of high-voltage waves, you can perform even the most difficult of tasks without burning out.

You do not need to do......

You do not
need to do
anything
other
than use
this flame
to invoke
the power of
consciousness
and then
repeat it
repeatedly

DNA

Step 24

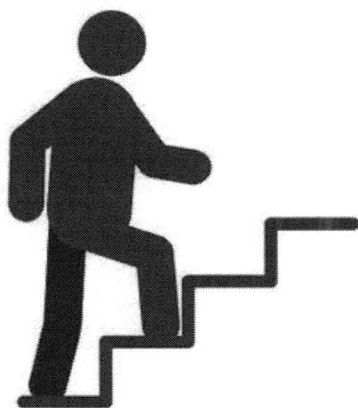

A way to disconnect for ultimate connection with Darvish Sufi Dance - Elevate your mind with this new paradigm

In next few pages you're about to find out!

- Let's find out about a state of mind far more powerful than sleep and wakefulness.

- What was the reason for Maulana Rumi's invention of Sufi dance? Does it have any mind-boosting properties?

- How can one spin in a circle 24 times a minute during the Sufi Dance of Dervishes? Like a planet, the flowing movements connect to the ultimate forces of the universe.

- Is there a scientific explanation for how Buddha reached Nirvana? Let's find out.

- What is the reason that spiritual experiences and situations cannot be described in words?

- What brainwave can take you to your deepest layers?

I always wanted to see whirling dervishes perform the mystical Sufi dance known as a sama, which involves a series of mesmerising turns as the Darvesh performs. In Istanbul, I was enchanted by the non-stop circular movement of the whirling Sufis, both clockwise and anticlockwise, that mesmerised me with its beauty. This is the first time I experienced this continuous rotation around one's axis and on a dance floor.

I found it impossible to believe this continuous rotation was possible without an intense flow state of mind. When witnessing that Sufi dance, my inner neurologist told me these Darvesh must be in a deep flow state. They could only be in such an extreme state of mind and body due to powerful waves flooding his brain. Each Darvesh was detached from the physical world, time, space, and any form of awareness or connection to the outside world.

In literal terms, "Darvesh" refers to a "doorway". In this sense, it signifies that a person himself can act as a bridge between two worlds—the materialistic world on the one hand and the heavenly spiritual world on the other.

As the dancer whirls (20-30 rotations per Minute), their brains are synchronised with theta rhythm, chanting Allah's name about 99 times a minute. Whirling is intended to give the dervish a sense of "emptying" himself of all distractions, which is the physiological and psychological purpose of the practice.

> I was enchanted by the non-stop circular movement of the whirling Sufis, both clockwise and anticlockwise, that mesmerised me with its beauty.

I found it impossible to......

I found it
impossible to
believe this
continuous rotation
was possible
without an intense
flow state of
mind. When
witnessing that
Sufi dance, my
inner neurologist
told me Darvish
was in a deep flow
state

DNA

"

What was the reason for Maulana Rum's invention of Sufi dance? Does it have any mind-boosting properties?

"

DNA

The famous mystic and poet Jalaluddin Rumi organised a spinning dervish ceremony to meditate as early as the 13th century. Rumi, born in Persia but lived in Konya then, was one of the greatest Sufis ever.

It is said that he told his followers that many avenues could lead to divinity and God. One path I suggest to you is that of dance and music. Rumi is famous for fasting, meditating, and dancing to achieve an enlightened state that is unparalleled in the world.

At this point, I would like to discuss the concept of Haal an exceptional state of mind. It is a temporary state of existence resulting from a Sufi's spiritual practices along his path towards God. The heart and soul are overwhelmed by a spiritual state. There are several spiritual states, and the perfect ones are beyond the description of words.

> At this point, I would like to discuss the concept of Haal's exceptional state of mind. It is a temporary state of existence resulting from a Sufi's spiritual practices

It is also defined as a Transcendent state of consciousness. What is it? It is an advanced state of consciousness believed to differ from waking, sleeping, and hypnotic states. It is a state of consciousness where a person can access higher levels of awareness and understanding. This can lead to spiritual growth, insight, and enhanced creativity and problem-solving.

There are many ways through which transcendental states can be attained, ranging from meditation, yoga, and prayer. Spiritual practices such as muraqba give us a greater sense of awareness, interconnectedness, the ability to find answers to complex questions and a deeper understanding of life's meaning. Mystical states, to me, are due to the deep state of the flow of the mind. Muraqba is a state of consciousness beyond the everyday

"

What was the reason for Maulana Rum's invention of Sufi dance? Does it have any mind-boosting properties?

"

DNA

experience of the physical world. It is a state of deep peace, bliss, and oneness, where one feels connected to everything. It is a state of pure joy and total acceptance.

The real questions are: can shifting brain waves result in "spiritual awakening"? Gamma brainwaves are usually very weak and uncommon in a common man. Mostly Tibetan Buddhists, martial art masters, highly elevated mystics, and ascended spiritual masters can vibrate at this frequency. This is the secret: if you are willing to have a spiritual awakening, you need these brain waves by immersing yourself in soul-searching activities.

This is the secret if you are **willing** to have a spiritual **awakening, you need** these brain waves by **immersing yourself** in soul-**searching** activities.

The "Parietal cortex" or "left inferior parietal lobule" is part of the brain that processes spiritual experiences. Also, when an individual becomes intensely aware of himself, this part of the brain is activated. A person's attention skills also stimulate it. Researchers referred to this portion of the brain as the "neurobiological home" of spiritual experience. This is activated whenever people experience a sense of connection that could feel overwhelmed with a power greater than themselves.

Now, I want to give you a perspective on Nirvana, the Enlightenment, that I hypothesise was achieved due to the deep flow state of mind that Buddha attained. The historical Buddha, also known as Gautama Buddha or Shakyamuni Buddha, is believed to have been about 29 years old when he embarked upon his quest for enlightenment.

Nearly six years after he began the search, in his mid-30s, he completed it. The man tortured himself, held his breath, and fasted to the point where he felt his ribs becoming stuck "like a spindle." He could almost feel his spine from his stomach. However, enlightenment did not seem to be on the horizon.

One day, he sat under the fig tree, and for the first time in his life, he entered a new realm of reality; that is, he was absorbed in a state of deep meditation. Sitting in the shade of the tree for six days and six nights, he realised that this experience was a stepping-stone leading to realisation. Instead of punishing his body to free himself from the bonds of the self, he will practice purity of mind and work with nature to realise enlightenment. To me, this was only possible due to the deep state of flow of mind.

Now I want to give you......

Now, I want to give you a perspective on Nirvana, the Enlightenment, that I hypothesise was achieved due to the deep flow state of Mind that Buddha attained.

DNA

Step 25

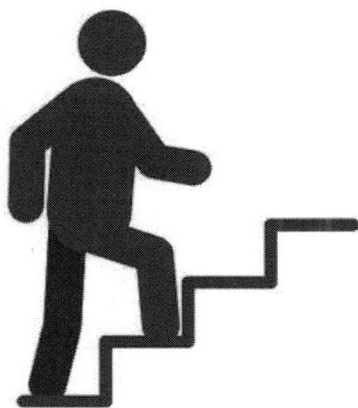

Think Like a Child and act like an adult - unlock your own creativity

In next few pages
you're about to find out!

- As we grow old, do we lose the sense of wonder and curiosity we once had as children? Do we know why?

- Could we be able to reclaim the power of imagination we had as children as we age?

- To realise our potential, does it make sense to see the world through the eyes of a child?

- Does there exist a reason why children do not have a time-scarcity mindset? In what ways can we apply the golden rule through the flow state?

- **What can children teach us about getting into a Flow State distinctively and seamlessly?**

There is a sense of wonder and curiosity about the world that we are filled with as children. In a child's world, no detail is too small to notice. We tend to lose our childlike sense of wonder, curiosity and the ability to see the world in new and different ways as we age.

The good news is that young imagination, curiosity, and creativity are still very much alive inside your mind – no matter how old you are. You will regain that mindset by getting flow states more often.

Children question almost everything they come across. If you ask them to be quiet on the bus, they will ask why? The question "Why" is used by every child to help guide their learning path. They only accept something once they can rationalise it and provide a rational and justifiable reason for taking it.

When we are young, our imagination is not limited by rules. When we are young, our vision is boundless. It is limitless and unbound to create our reality, free to develop our thinking style. We could quickly and easily get into a state of flow during our childhood.

Let me tell you about exciting research in which questions were posed to two groups of North Dakota State University college students regarding what they would do on a day off. One group was instructed to think like a seven-year-old, and the other group was prepared to accept anything as an adult.

> The good news is that young imagination, curiosity, and creativity are still very much alive inside your mind — no matter how old you are

When we are young......

When we
are young, our
imagination is
not Limited by
rules. When we
are young, our
vision is
boundless. It is
Limitless
and unbound to
create our
reality

DNA

"

As we grow older, do we lose the sense of wonder and curiosity we once had as children? Do we know why?

"

DNA

This experiment was conducted with hundreds of students, and the results were consistent. The groups instructed to think like a child consistently developed more creative and innovative solutions.

In other words, feel like a child if you want to be more creative. Apple's CEO, Steve Jobs, brought a childlike questioning genius to the field of product design. A youthful instinct to create one of the world's best-selling products. As adults, we consider the world full of obstacles, but as children, we don't. During your journey, there was a time when you felt belittled and stopped believing in your own abilities. Your belief in possibilities used to be strong, but now you think things are impossible.

> As adults, we consider the world full of obstacles, but as children, we don't. During your journey, there was a time when you felt belittled and stopped believing in your own abilities

Here is why we change as adults. The reason is as our frontal lobes grow with age; more perceptions and limitations begin to grasp onto the reins of our minds. The child truly believes that they can achieve anything; the child feels that they can become a pilot, a doctor, an astronaut, a president, or any idea that comes to the child's mind. A child's world is full of endless possibilities for them.

A child isn't afraid to change their mind when they are made to. Sadly, as adults, we tend to believe that sticking to a decision or one course of action is a sign of maturity, which presents a significant obstacle if we need to change course.

The results of studies show that having a time-scarcity mindset can significantly affect your well-being. This is an ironic perspective because the more successful you become, the more likely you are

"

What can children
teach us about
getting into a Flow
State distinctively
and seamlessly?

"

DNA

to fall into this mindset. Considering that most children do not entirely comprehend the concept of time, this results in them not feeling pressured by a theoretical time limit. When doing a task, try not to pay attention to the time.

If you were to watch children playing, what would you notice about them? They are entirely absorbed in what they are doing. If you call their names and try to get their attention, you will find that only some will not respond. The reason for this is that they are in a flow state. Their game is so good because they are immersed in it. As a result, they are unwilling to come out of it. They are happily absorbed in it. The bubble of flow state keeps the kids interested, and they will not get bored quickly in this environment.

The flow state makes children willing to learn anything, and they don't consider anything complex. This process of the flow state is embedded in our minds from childhood. As we grow older, however, we gradually remove this process from our minds. There are many ways to reinstall them correctly, but we must rekindle the child within us.

The result of......

The results of
studies show
that having a time-
scarcity mindset
can significantly
affect your
well-being.
This is an ironic
perspective
because the more
successful you
become, the
more likely
you are to
fall into this
mindset

DNA

Step 26

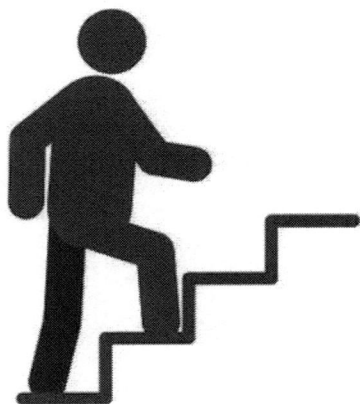

Intuition - Acquire the art of making intuitive learning and decision-making faster

In next few pages
you're about to find out!

- Which person has given the greatest theory in the history of humankind by believing in his intuition?

- What is the mechanism by which the brain acquires information for us without our knowledge?

- What is the best way to turn on the brain switch of intuition?

- How do you connect with your brain's intuitive network?

- It is a good idea to ask intuition a question, but why?

- Imagine what would happen if you started using and believing in your sixth sense

- Take some time to think alone among the trees.

Intuitive people generate ideas and make decisions without much deliberate thinking about them. Understanding intuition involves thinking and acting without being explicitly prompted by the conscious mind.

Intuition is a skill anyone can develop over time through a process that I call "Thirst and Training". In this process, you must first allow yourself to crave intuitive hints from the cosmic intelligence network. Observe the world around and within you.

I think it would be prudent sometimes to give rest to your logical mind and give space to your intuitive mind on your mind screen. Let your deepest instincts of wisdom rise to the surface at times. By the use of flow, these ideas could be telecasted to your brilliant mind.

I am pleased to share this exciting news. We can obtain extremely high levels of intuitive access. However, this power of the mind has remained hidden behind closed doors. Our intuitive thoughts can start coming to us in small increments if we practice the flow of the mind and exercise regularly. When we can access flow states, we can receive information transcending space and time.

Let's see how we can make this work. The first step is to desire intuition and train our minds to obtain information from the subconscious. It is a process of absorbing information

> **Intuition is a skill anyone can develop over time through a process that I call "Thirst and Training". In this process, you must first allow yourself to crave intuitive hints from the cosmic intelligence network**

I am pleased to share......

I am pleased
to share this
exciting
news. We can
obtain
extremely
high Levels
of intuitive
access.
However, this
power of the
mind has
remained
hidden behind
closed doors

DNA

"

What is the
mechanism by which
the brain acquires
information for us
without our
knowledge?

"

DNA

from the environment around us without being aware of it.

In other words, when we seek intuitive abilities, and our minds know that we are seeking an intuitive path, our known and unknown brain sensors start developing connections, patterns, and relationships between the things we see or do not see consciously.

In turn, this information is used to generate alternatives and possibilities. It is no secret that Einstein was one of the most remarkable men in history. He was one of the most intelligent person to ever exist on the surface of the planet. He used his intuitive skills to solve challenging mathematical problems. . His ideas and theories are still studied and used in science today.

As soon as we face life challenges, our minds can imagine new scenarios and can almost immediately come up with various options. If a door closes, a favourable frame intuition will open multiple doors for you.

> It is a process of absorbing information from the environment around us without being aware of it. In other words, when we seek intuitive abilities and our minds know that we are seeking an intuitive path

Do you see how many possibilities exist? As there are so many options to consider, it can be hard to rationally explain why people feel stuck when so many opportunities are available, feeling as if they have no options without recognising them.

It is through a flow that possibilities are created. In this way, you'll be taken into new dimensions in pursuing new ideas, potentials, and opportunities that have yet to be thought of. Spend time daily in solitude if you wish to be intuitive.

Give the topic of self-consultation to your mind gently, and then let the ideas come on to your screen of consciousness without searching for them. You feel brilliant thoughts are like butterflies, coming to you as you choose. Could you imagine yourself without limitations or boundaries? What would you do if you could?

Let me ask, can you do what you want? Imagine being surrounded by the positive vibrations of positive thoughts and images. As you sink into the depths of your deeper self, an inner bridge forms, leading you to your higher self. If you close your eyes, you will experience this. It would help if you wrote down what you experienced afterwards. Now let me ask you at this stage and leave you with food for thought. Could you make that vivid image a reality?

> Imagine being surrounded by the positive vibrations of positive thoughts and images.
> As you sink into the depths of your deeper self, an inner bridge forms, leading you to your higher self.

Let me share this fascinating real-life sport of shooting a moving target instead of a fixed one while riding a horse at a fast pace called horse archery. During the shot, the archer and the target had moved relative to each other, further complicating the situation. As a horse rider galloping at top speed while on top of a horse, it is almost impossible to shoot using only the eyes.

For this reason, intuitive shooting techniques are critical to mounted archery. An intuitive ability to calculate speed and distance is necessary for riders to reach their target using muscle memory and hand-eye coordination.

Due to this technique, an archer can shoot while keeping both eyes

"

What is the best way to turn on the brain switch of intuition?

"

DNA

fixed on the target throughout the entire execution of the shot.

Can you consider yourself that if an archer could use intuitive skills, why can't you in a fast-moving, challenging life?

Researchers designed an experiment that exposed participants to emotional images as they attempted to make an accurate decision to measure intuition. Researchers found that even when participants were unaware of the pictures, they could still make more precise and confident decisions based on the information from the images. During the experiment, college students were shown a moving cloud of dots, like what you might see on an old television.

The participants had to report whether the cloud of dots was moving left or right. When they made their sensory judgments, they were presented with emotional photographs. While making decisions, researchers used techniques to make inspirational pictures barely visible or unconscious to them. Images included positive and negative images, including a snake about to strike and adorable puppies.

A study found that people made faster and more accurate decisions when they unconsciously viewed pictures that evoked strong positive emotions. It was found that people's brains could process and utilise information from images to improve their decision-making abilities. In addition, another interesting finding from this study was that intuition improved over time, suggesting that the mechanisms of intuition can be enhanced with practice. According to the study, we can use unconscious information in our bodies and brains to help guide us through life, enabling better, faster, and more confident decisions.

As a child, I clearly remember my father Sehba Akhtar having a keen sense of intuition. I am still trying to determine from where it originated. I believe that my father's intuition was something that he developed over time and through some inner and deeper experience., I believe that it was his poetic mindset that made it possible. It was a bridge of poetic flow, allowing ideas to come to him rather than him chasing them. During the process practised over decades, the cosmic intelligence network up in the skies, combined with his deep, hidden, intuitive network, offered him ideas on an intuitive level. Based on that, he could predict things and anticipate things and make decisions based on that.

As a child, I clearly remember......

As a child, I
clearly remember
my father Sehba
Akhtar having a
keen sense of
intuition. I am still
trying to determine
from where it
originated

DNA

Step 27

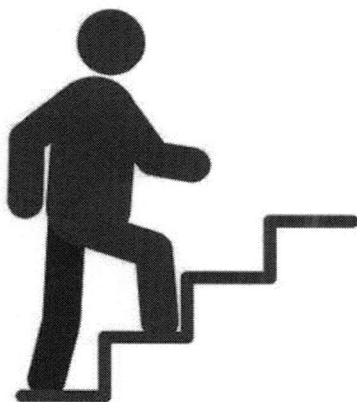

How to utilise impact of your room on your thinking, Creating a creative and productive environment?

In next few pages you're about to find out!

- In your life, where do you spend the most of your time?

- There is so much more to your room than just walls and ceilings that you should make it yours.

- Your room's walls and doors can transmit the most powerful messages to you

- What is the importance of the room being bright, colourful, smelling good, hearing good, and having a good view?

- Your living room needs a living, breathing plant.

- There should always be three books next to your bed in your room.

All the Visual cues must help you supercharge your brain waves to trigger the flow state. Every image that catches your eye drives energy. It will help if you have an energised environment. The energy sources that I would like to arrange in my room, whether they are candles or inspirational pictures, are things that I would like to be there. An energy source is what makes it possible for us to function.

A natural presence can be experienced through the five senses and more. To me It is a myth that we have only five senses. We do not even question it because it's so accepted as fact.

Flow state triggers are there in the environment; if it is your room and you are connected to a chair and a table, you need the scene in front of you now. Keep working on the triggers of the flow state. It is said that picture depicts a story of one thousand words. True, but sometimes some images even can carry million vivid words and intense meanings to your mind that one can ignite a slow volcano of energy.

Secondly, if you can choose colours and lighting in the room, try to have a dim blue light somewhere around you. There should be some light music around you.

A cluttered workspace means a distracted mind. Abraham Maslow was the first to work on the theory of motivation and describe the human hierarchy of needs. His experiments were fascinating and

> All the Visual cues must help you supercharge your brain waves to trigger the flow state. Every image that catches your eye drives energy

321

Flow state triggers......

Flow state
triggers are
there in the
environment; if
it is your room
and you are
connected to a
chair and a
table

DNA

"

In your Life, where do you spend the most of your time?

"

DNA

intelligent. Is there a connection between the environment and the human psyche?

As a result of his wife and colleagues' assistance, three rooms were built at the university. The first room consists of a cosy chair with various artwork, a bookshelf, and a precious rug decorated with an array of precious stones. It is referred to as a beautiful room. The other room was decorated as an average room, and the third room was highly cluttered with random items, many of which contained empty boxes. The ashtrays were scattered throughout the room, and all the furniture and items were arranged in a random manner.

> The brain registers all the visual information around us; whether we look at it attentively or inadvertently

Then a group of different students were sent to these three rooms, and these students were to look at some pictures and give them numbers on energy and well-being on a numerical scale, i.e., images with power and well-being. They were asked to look at them and give them numbers from 1 to 5. You will be surprised to know that the group of students who were in the beautiful room, when they saw the pictures related to well-being and energy, scored more, that is, gave more marks. However, when the same pictures were shown to the students in the next room, they saw the same images and scored low marks.

Undoubtedly, our aesthetic satisfaction is essential for our energy production. The brain registers all the visual information around us; whether we look at it attentively or inadvertently, Maslow discovered this and then presented it to the world. Let me say this here. If you want to invest:

- Save money and make your living room beautiful.

- Post pictures of people whose company can impress you.

- Decorate your walls with quotes that make your brain register this message repeatedly.

> **Keep in mind that whatever you see around you. It also takes up a space in your mind and brain**

When the last prophet of God said that cleanliness is half faith, the science of psychology made it clear that our mental and emotional health has much to do with organization and cleanliness. A wealth of research shows how light intensity, sound intensity, and colours in a room affect our children's learning and how each person's cognitive thinking ideas can affect continuity and flow. Keep in mind whatever you see around you. It also takes up space in your mind, in your brain, clutter can cause mental chaos. All the visual cues must help you supercharge your brain waves to trigger the flow state. Every image that catches your eye drives energy. It will help if you have an energised environment.

Make sure you buy some plants for your room. Plants can purify the air and reduce stress. They can also add a touch of greenery and freshness to your room. Plants can add a sense of comfort and cosiness. According to NASA, some indoor plants improve the quality of air inside and make the study space more relaxing. Moreover, plants can also help reduce stress levels and create a more inviting atmosphere.

It is a good idea to turn off your phone if you live in your specific study area. You should not put this in your pocket. The best thing to do is to turn it off or at least switch it to aeroplane mode. You can find that your phone can be one of your biggest distractions while you are reading. If you do not expect an important call, turn your phone off whenever you sit down to study so that you have a mental break.

Buy some plants......

Buy some plants.
NASA has proven
that some indoor
plants improve
indoor air quality,
and some green and
living things make
the study space
calmer. If you live
in your specific
study area

DNA

Step 28

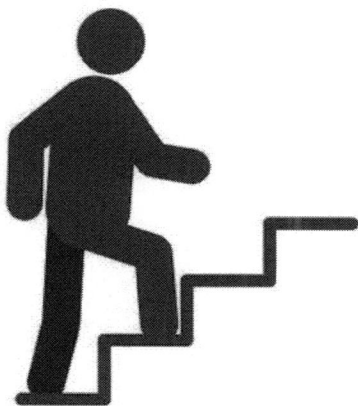

The magical effects of music on the brain - How to use music to boost your brain waves

In next few pages
you're about to find out!

- Is it true that everything in the universe is always in flux?

- What can we gain by knowing that every particle of our body has a flow within it?

- How much power is there in music and tones? Through his music and raga, Tansen made it rain and lit up the extinguished Lamps, but how?

- What are the findings of a study on the brains of 9,000 musicians?

- What is the mechanism by which the sound of music activates the powerful waves of our mind?

No matter what it is in this universe. vibration and motion make up its existence. Everything in the universe is in motion. The survival of life can be seen as a music note hidden within a specific frequency. Our entire body is made up of atoms in motion. We can get into the most powerful state with the mental flow.

When it comes to the history of South Asian music, Tansen holds the highest throne in terms of his contributions. History suggests that TanSen used to induce rain with his music. He is reputed to have caused rainfall by singing a Raga called Meg Malhar (rain song) and lighting up the lamps by singing a Raga called Deepak (Fire Raga). It may never be known how many facts are in it and how much truth this historic narration contains.

However, one thing is sure: music is a great invention of man, and this invention has allowed humanity to express their happiness and to entertain and soothe themselves.

There is scientific evidence to support this. When you listen to music, you are not only elated with your emotions, but you can also experience a state of mental flow due to the chemical and electrical changes in your brain caused by it. To get into a state of flow, some music enthusiasts repeatedly listen to the same favourite song. They can't stop listening to it. As a result of listening to this, they will be able to achieve mental equanimity. There is also a lot of research on this.

> No matter what it is in this universe. vibration and motion make up its existence. Everything in the universe is in motion. The survival of life can be seen as a music note hidden within a specific frequency. Our entire body is made up of atoms in motion

History suggests that......

History suggests
that TanSen used
to induce rain
with his music. He
is reputed to have
caused rainfall by
singing a Raga
called Meg
Malhar
(rain song)
and lighting up
the lamps by
singing a Raga
called Deepak
(Fire Raga)

DNA

"

Is it true that everything in the universe is always in flux? "

DNA

Let me give you an example to make a piece of music resonate in your mind. Ton-Ton-Ton-Ton-Ton-Ton-Ton. Try to hear it in your mind. Check it out how do you feel while imagining this piece of tune in your mind. Now try and imagine La-La-Laa-La. You can feel the difference it makes on your mind.

A major study on 9,000 brain wave samples of musician's brains found that musicians were twice as capable of thinking and focusing their thoughts on a single point due to certain powerful electrical waves generated in the brain caused by music. The electrical waves begin to take hold, and the flow in the brain taking the brain out of anxious waves and converting them into powerful alpha waves. A powerful and electric fortress

> **A major** study on **9,000 brain wave** samples **found that** musicians **were twice as capable of thinking and** focusing **their thoughts on a single** point **due to certain powerful electrical**

of alpha waves is built. And unnecessary ideas from outside cannot enter inside it.

The abilities to learn and understand are multiplied. Further question is whether music is a powerful source of mental energy as well, what the research says. Let me tell you about a sound technique called binaural beats. If Two tones of slightly different frequencies are played simultaneously in different ears using headphones creates a new third tone, which has a frequency equal to that difference between the two tones. This auditory illusion is called a binaural beat. For example, if a person hears a tone of 105 Hz in one ear and a tone of 115 Hz in the other, they will hear a binaural beat with a frequency of 10 Hz.

While your conscious mind won't be able to detect the difference

"

What can we gain by knowing that every particle of our body has a flow within it?

"

DNA

between the beats, your brain will be able to, and because of the exposure to the beats, your brain's operation will change. Listening to them has been scientifically proven to increase our focus many times. it sweeps away all anxieties and scattered imaginations that stand in its way and opens the door to new possibilities.

Neuroscience has shown that music triggers your emotions and changes your mind chemically and electrically. There is no doubt that it will have the desired effect of bringing you into a state of mental flow. Many people listen to the same favourite song repeatedly to achieve this magical state of mental flow. Several studies have indicated that listening to it can help you achieve mental alignment.

Neuroscience has shown **that** **music** triggers your **emotions** **and changes** your mind **chemically** and electrically. I **bring that** which can **work** **to bring you** **into a state** of mental flow

Let me tell you......

Let me tell you
about a sound
technique called
binaural beats. If
Two tones of
slightly different
frequencies are
played
simultaneously in
different ears
using
headphones creates
a new
third tone

DNA

Step 29

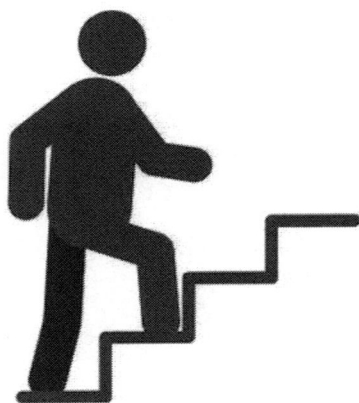

How shower can instigate brilliant ideas – learn the trick

In next few pages you're about to find out!

- You probably don't know that you have slow, fast, and super-fast tracks of thinking. Do you?

- How can the slow, fast, and super-fast brain pathways of thinking can be used?

- What other surprising changes does taking a shower make to the surface of our brains that we can use for our ideas?

- What was the Archimedes Eureka moment? And how can we create eureka moments in our lives?

- How can Aqua Notes be used while bathing?

- How and why does a new idea suddenly jump to the surface of the mind while taking a shower? How can we use it in our practical life?

To think faster and create insight networks more quickly, there is a fast track and a super-fast track. It is when a solution or novel idea appears out of nowhere in your head. This phenomenon is known as the "aha" moment and is a sign of creativity, insight, and intelligence.

Both the fast track and the super-fast path offer substantial potential for quick thinking and creating networks of intelligence; however, it is imperative to remember that the slow track can still be beneficial. A state of flow will magically trigger your fast-track thinking. To ensure success, it is important to strike a balance between the fast and slow tracks and to stay in the flow.

This is an interesting example that I would like to share with you. It demonstrates how we can find connections between different pieces of information and use them to our advantage. How can taking a shower or being in the bath flash an idea by stimulating the fast track of our thinking rather than the slow one? This example highlights how a seemingly mundane task like taking a shower or bath can stimulate creative ideas and lead to creative solutions. This is because it taps into the fast track of our thinking.

One of the greatest mathematicians of antiquity was Archimedes. His most famous story is that of King Hieron II of Syracuse and the gold crown. As a

To think faster and create insight networks more quickly, there is a fast track and a super fast path. It is when a solution or novel idea appears out of nowhere in your head

tribute to the gods, the King commissioned the creation of a crown. A smith produced a beautiful crown from carefully weighed gold.

Shower or bath can stimulate......

This example
highlights
how a
seemingly
mundane task
like taking a
shower or
bath can
stimulate
creative ideas
and lead to
creative
solutions

DNA

"

You probably don't
know that you
have slow, fast,
and super-fast
tracks of thinking.
Do you?

"

DNA

tribute to the gods, the King commissioned the creation of a crown.

A smith produced a beautiful crown from carefully weighed gold. Nevertheless, the King became suspicious that the craftsman still needed to use all the gold he had been given. To solve the problem, he turned to his close friend Archimedes.

As Archimedes knew, gold and silver weigh differently, so gold weighs about twice as much as silver. The problem was that people needed help to figure out

> **Archimedes jumped out of the bath and ran naked down the streets, shouting, "Eureka!" — "I've found it!"**

how to work out the size of an irregularly shaped object like a crown because they needed to learn how to do that.

As Archimedes pondered this problem, he went to the public baths to relax and contemplate the solution. The moment he slipped into the water, he noticed some spilling of water over the edge, and inspiration struck him. There must be an exact match between him and the displaced water. Calculating an object's density is easy if you know its volume.

Archimedes had figured out whether a lump of pure gold with the same volume as the crown would weigh more than pure gold. The crown would have been lighter if the craftsman had used silver instead of gold. In a wild jubilation, Archimedes jumped out of the bath and ran naked down the streets, shouting, "Eureka!" - "I've found it!".

When you are in the shower, especially if you have been thinking, your ideas can be woken up from their "incubation period". Your subconscious mind has been working to solve your problems, and you don't even know it. Taking a shower is like watering seeds, as seeds grow when they are watered. Similarly, ideas grow and surface in our minds when we shower.

"

How and why does a
new idea suddenly
jump to the surface
of the mind while
taking a shower? How
can we use it in our
practical life?

"

DNA

Zero to Volcano - 33 Steps to Superstate of your Magical Mind
by DNA

After we get into the shower, the falling water unleashes ideas from our awakened brain as soon as we step in. We suddenly get a flood of ideas, and our mind is clear as a result. Why does this happen?

Creative thunder occurs, and a new insight appears suddenly and magically, and we break our mental barriers. A flow state can explicitly explain these Eureka and Aha Moments.

Let me explain. Your brain can solve problems in two different ways. It is possible to approach problems logically, i.e., systematically, and deliberately think of possible solutions. Furthermore, you have a fast track of thinking, a super-fast path that enables you to learn quickly. It's a faster way to discover answers than systematically approaching the problem, resulting in an Aha! Moment. it is an incredibly rewarding experience that can save time and effort.

There is now a question about the Neuroscientific secret for activating the flow state in the shower. If we were to answer, perhaps, we would say that when we shower, I believe the water that falls on our heads creates alpha waves, then cold water causes our dopamine and cannabinoid levels to go high. This results in lateral thinking and combining different thoughts to generate novel ideas.

For those who like to think while in the shower, Aqua Notes may be of interest. Aqua Notes is a waterproof notepad that sticks to the wall of the shower. It allows users to jot down their ideas without having to worry about getting the notepad wet. It's perfect for those who like to brainstorm in the shower.

Especially in the morning and especially if you can get a cold shower, be sure to think in the shower and get clever ideas. Keep a notebook with you when you are in the shower. To my colleagues, I also say, in a light-hearted way, that if you take a shower and return without clever ideas, it has been a waste of water.

Be sure to think in the......

Be sure to
think in the
shower and get clever
ideas Keep a notebook
with you when
you are in the shower,
I also say, in a light-
hearted way,
that if you
take a shower and
return without
an idea or clever
ideas, it has been a
waste of water

DNA

Step 30

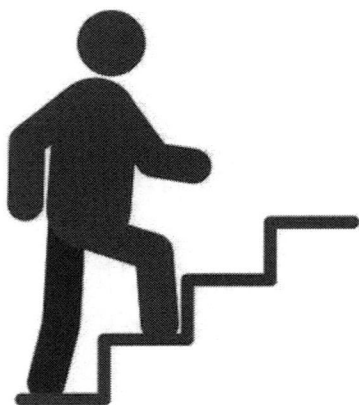

How to use the super power of collective consciousness?

In next few pages you're about to find out!

- What is "C" energy that can be found in libraries or other places where people engage in collective thinking?

- What is a 3C phenomenon, according to me? By understanding this, you can create an optimal electromagnetic environment for your brain.

- How does our brain's default setting work?

- **How do focused people create an energised environment around them?**

I have been wondering for years whether libraries have an electromagnetic wave spectrum that affects our brains, and I have been thinking about this hypothesis for a long time. My theory is based on the simple concept that a place where many people sit together and concentrate generates a field of energy spread throughout the room.

I strongly believe whenever people focus collectively, even on different ideas and topics, they create an undiscovered form of energy. This environment allows you to share, upload, and download energy. This energy can be used to generate creativity and innovation, leading to amazing discoveries and solutions. This energy is contagious; it spreads to the environment and opens new paths and opportunities.

There is a palpable aura of "collective concentrating consciousness". A three-C phenomenon is what I call it. I am curious to know how many more decades it will take to prove this hypothesis, but why not explore the collective impact of focused mind energies instead of waiting?

Can I ask if you could explain to me why you are unable to focus on your studies in the same way you were able to do in a library?

I believe that the one thing that unequivocally matters is the environment in which we live. As far as the library environment is concerned, it is a peaceful, calm place

> I have been wondering for years whether libraries have an electromagnetic wave spectrum that affects our brains, and I have been thinking about this hypothesis for a long time.

There is a palpable aura ......

There is a
palpable aura of
"collective
concentrating
consciousness". A
three-C
phenomenon is
what I call it.

DNA

"

What is "C" energy that can be found in Libraries or other places where people engage in collective thinking?

"

DNA

where people are also studying simultaneously, which motivates us. This is to inform the mind that it is in a study area. We did not come here to sleep, eat, or drink but to learn. As soon as you do this, it becomes effortless for you to concentrate.

Our subconscious mind is the key to this. A default setting in our brain is imprinted as early as childhood. When you walk into a mosque, you think of praying; when you walk into a field, you envision playing; when you enter a bedroom, you fantasise about relaxing; and when you enter a theatre, you imagine watching movies. Likewise, when you think of libraries, your mind immediately brings to mind the process of focusing.

> Our subconscious mind is the key to this. A default setting in our brain is imprinted as early as childhood

You can focus more if you have a proper study table. Have a dedicated study schedule where you are not disturbed.

Most functional magnetic resonance imaging (fMRI) studies are conducted with the subject lying in the supine position, which has been discussed as a potential confounding factor in such studies. It has been suggested that cognitive functions, such as problem-solving and perception, will differ between supine and upright positions. Studies have confirmed that, in contrast to a slumped posture, an upright seated posture can enhance positive mood, reduce negative mood, and maintain self-esteem. Upright seated posture increases speech rates.

Studies have confirmed that ......

Studies have
confirmed that,
in contrast to
slumped posture, an
upright seated
posture can enhance
positive mood, reduce
negative mood, and
maintain self-esteem.
Upright seated
posture increases
speech rates.

DNA

Step 31

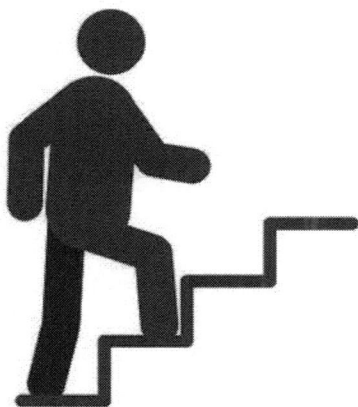

Four super power stages to your mystical flow

In next few pages you're about to find out!

- What four important stages are necessary to bring us into mental flow?

- You must use your mind in a certain way. Let's find out next.

- How not to build dams in front of flowing ideas.

- How to stop the newscaster of your mind?

- **Why is it important to keep the flame of emotions low in mental flow?**

First stage

We must set a goal for ourselves as the first stage in achieving the Flow state. It is imperative to understand that the flow state is not an aimless state. There is no such thing as being in an empty-minded flow state. In the flow state, physical and mental activity is directed towards a goal.

Even though it is essential to set a goal for ourselves after doing this, we should focus on completing the steps that will lead us to our destination. Every aspect of one's being is devoted to the steps to the extent that the whole of one's existence is immersed in them. This leads to a sense of unity between the task and yourself. Ultimately, you become one with the task.

As soon as you have set your goal, you will focus on the steps that will lead you towards achieving it, whether a learning or a physical task, creative or related to daily life activities. There is no margin for you to pay attention to anything else, not even the target itself since the present step requires your undivided attention. The task will be easier for you if you thoroughly understand it.

To achieve this goal, you must know well what steps to take. Let me refer to what Einstein said: we must first learn the game's rules and then play better than anyone else. It is prudent to assume that every step becomes the most significant step in your life as you face this challenge.

> We must set a goal for ourselves as the first step in getting to the Flow state. It is imperative to understand that the flow state is not an aimless state.

363

"

What four important steps are necessary to bring us into mental flow?

"

DNA

First, you must decide which life challenge you want to understand. After that, you have to get involved with it. You mustn't leave this topic to ensure that this flow state lasts for half an hour to an hour. It would help if you did not even ponder when this state ends. Every step is a "Happy Journey of Internal Flow" towards attaining the desired target and fulfilling every possible goal.

Let me refer to what Einstein said: we must first learn the game's rules and then play better than anyone else

There are means and methods that can be used to manage our minds to achieve our objectives. Some strategies can guide and trigger the mind's inherent powers for it to behave in a specific way. Slipping into the flow of the mind is known as "slipping into the zone". A supercharged electrochemical state can take place in your brain. As soon as you adopt this method, you unknowingly slip into the flow state. You will be so lost in your task that you don't even realise you have achieved it.

Stage 2

Flow with the Flow

You need to select a topic that interests you, a problem you wish to solve, and a topic you want to learn, and then decide what you want to generate mentally and what you wish to create. After you've figured that out, ideas will start flowing. In a state of mental flow, you must let these thoughts flow. These thoughts don't need to be examined for quality. Critique is not necessary. It would be best to allow your thoughts to stream on your mind's screen. It is important not to view this activity as an end but rather to

A supercharged electrochemical......

A
supercharged
electrochemical
state can take
place in your
brain. As soon as
you adopt this
method, you
unknowingly slip
into the
flow state
without
knowing it.

DNA

achieve an end. Due to this, it should not be used to determine when the flow state will end. Every statement that you make in your mind flows effortlessly with your thoughts. To be able to experience flow would be one of the most rewarding feelings one could encounter in one's life. They are disassociated from all distractions, sinking into the ideal peak mental state they could achieve.

This is a process of inner evolution as your mind will be revealing what you do not expect to come from yourself. A pleasant surprise for you from your deeper self. You will be amazed to know that the inner conflicting battle of thoughts has been resolved, an idea is about to emerge, and a question that has been mishandled is about to be answered.

Stage 3

Switch off Minds Newscaster

Society has conditioned us to read and listen to sensational news, gossip, unappealing headlines, and breaking news across all media platforms. To put it another way, we are in a constant state of searching for such information. As a result of mind programming, we are constantly directed to listen to and read these things. Similarly, our mind acts as a newscaster continuously broadcasting numerous news items.

The problem is that it keeps bringing new news to our attention regularly. News from yesterday, news from today, news of people's attitudes, and perhaps even news from tomorrow. To achieve flow, you must switch off your mind's newscaster before and during a flow state. We need to regain the role of the master controller of our minds, like that of an editor of a news channel. Editors are responsible for editing the news flow, as they must oversee the flow of communication. You should be able to determine which information should be forwarded to your mind and which should be ignored and discarded entirely.

To achieve the state of flow in your mind, you must shut down your own inner news channel and its newscaster. There is no doubt that

"

Why is it important to keep the flame of emotions low in mental flow?

"

DNA

the electric flow state is the most powerful state of mind we will be able to achieve when it comes to achieving our goals. I am sure that we will succeed.

Stage 4

Keep a low flame

When you are in a flow state, you will experience a particular emotional flow. But when entering this realm, it is essential to remember that the candle of emotions is burning within you. This is your emotional flame. The flame should have a unique level that should be set, so keep it flowing for a long duration. Low flame means the flame won't increase, so you can have candle of creativity shining within you for a long time. The candle wax would inevitably melt away if you had a high flame.

Flame cannot be dimmed too much since if they were dimmed too much, there would not be enough inner illumination. Like a dimly lit candle cannot illuminate a room, dimly lit ideas cannot enlighten your mind. Allow enlightened ideas to develop along with emotional stability and perseverance. I promise you will be surprised again by such great ideas that come with pride. When this zone is in this state, some people feel happy. There is a cannabinoid effect that comes with this unique flow of mind.

When you are in the......

When you are
in a flow state,
you will
experience a
particular
emotional
flow. But when
entering this
realm, it is
essential to
remember that the
candle of
emotions is
burning within
you.

DNA

Step 32

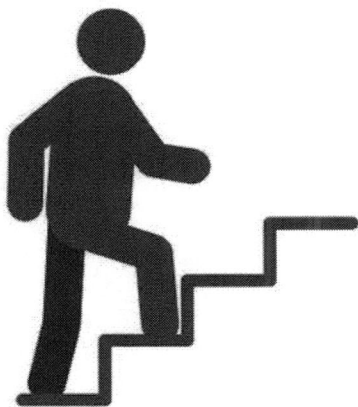

Supercharge your brain by learning breathing patterns?

In next few pages you're about to find out!

- How can the brain be supercharged in five seconds or so? Let's learn together.

- A new way of breathing is possible. What are the ways in which breathing can change the way we think and feel?

- What are the two wires (nerves) in your chest that control your breathing and potentially thinking? Let's know the secret.

You must have heard of meditation, and you must have some opinions about it. Many people consider it an unimportant exercise, and many are terrified of the word maraqba, as if it is the practice only for Sufi faqirs or philosophers. This concept is not entirely true. Everyone deserves to experience the same transcended state of mind and such a transformation is attainable for all, regardless of circumstances.

Muraqba is the spiritual practice of deep inner meditation, which can lead to a profound connection with the Divine and to a state of inner peace and serenity. It is believed to be an effective way to transform the mind and heart, leading to an awareness of the divine unity of all things. Muraqba can be utilised as a tool to achieve a state of flow to find solutions to the problems that face us in our daily life.

At this point, I want to introduce you to a new concept of Mini-Meditations which are exercises you can do for five seconds or less. Although you may need to become more familiar with the term, I use it myself, and the exercise I have prepared will help you get into the flow state. Instead of fast-paced brain waves, the electrical circuits of your brain must be converted into alpha waves if you want to transform your thinking into a robust flow state.

> **Muraqba can, however, be utilised as a tool to achieve a state of flow to find solutions to the problems that face us in our daily life.**

How long does it take to take a deep breath? A micro-meditation exercise involves taking a deep breath for five to ten seconds and focusing on it. Imagine your chest is being filled with freshness

Muraba is the spiritual......

Muraqba is the
spiritual
practice of inner
meditation,
which can
lead to a
profound
connection
with the Divine
and to a state
of inner peace
and serenity

DNA

"

How can the brain be supercharged in five seconds or so ? Let's Learn together.

"

DNA

and fresh air. Once you are comfortable and hear your breathing for a long time without any difficulty, try to introduce a mantra. A mantra is a recurring, word or a vocalisation that helps you focus.

During your meditation session, repeat your mantra over and over again. You can say a simple word "ho" at each exhale. When you breathe in, the thoughts will try to come back to your mind, and you need to focus only on a breath and sound of Ho.

I am confident that repeating these exercises repeatedly for five to ten seconds will calm your personality, and creative thoughts will return.

You can strengthen your brain's software system for focus by diverting your attention to your breath when you feel lost. When we recognise that we are off track or distracted by a text message or our phone, we can get back on track more quickly. If you lose your focus during the day, take a short meditation break. The following exercise can be used as a form of micro-meditation. Let a wave of relaxation wash over you from your toes to your head as if it were a wave of water. It passes through your whole existence and then back up again.

Stress is better handled by people who meditate. Research has shown that the amygdala - the part of the brain that responds to anxiety - calms down with meditation. A meditator can handle high-pressure situations with a lighter touch. This allows them to remain calm, focused and in control, even when the stakes are high.

I am confident that repeating these exercises for five to ten seconds will calm your personality, and creative thoughts will return. According to the research behind it, it has been found that the participant became active in several areas of his brain. A meditative practice performed before seeking an answer to a curious question reduces the time spent searching for an answer. You will become accustomed to fast thinking by performing these exercises. Regular practice lets you quickly identify the best solution to your queries, making the whole process of thinking much more efficient. Another study found that such exercises, which lasted from five to twenty-five seconds, reduced stress levels and increased hippocampus size, our brain's memory storage house, significantly.

You can strengthen......

You can
strengthen
your brain's
software system
for focus by
diverting your
attention
to your breath
when you
feel lost

DNA

Step 33

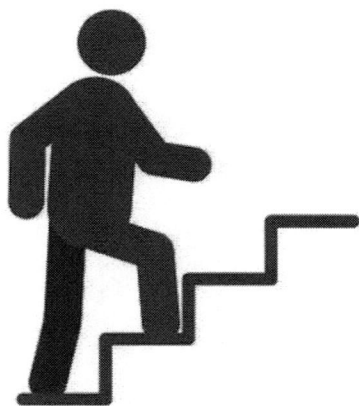

Flow zone
Exercises

In next few pages you're about to find out!

- Can we use our minds and our minds as we want?

- Who is your brain's supreme commander? How does it rule our minds? Let's understand this secret easily.

- How can you install new software in your mind?

- How can you convert the information and information your brain receives into ideas?

- Write on the paper with both hands simultaneously. What revolutionary change will it bring?

- In your imagination, visualise what you see by turning it clockwise direction upside down. What changes will it cause in the brain?

- What is the scientific secret to self-talk?

- On white unlined paper, write spontaneously. Brainstorming is a skill you should learn.

- The junction between sleep and wakefulness

- You have wasted your most precious time of the day since you were born,

so it's no wonder why you are so
easily distracted.

- The iron ball was held by Edison
  and other geniuses before they went
  to sleep. Why did they do this?

- How should one use the powerful
  waves of the mind immediately after
  waking up?

Super easy exercises can make anyone at any age brainier. As a first step, I want to reiterate what I stated in the previous chapter. The most valuable asset humans possess is taken from them without their knowledge. It is their attention span. Various studies show that the average person now has a brief attention span and cannot concentrate for long periods.

Let me ask a question: can we voluntarily focus our minds on a desired task, and if so, how long can we do so? Is it possible to stop our brains from doing something that interests us but is not necessarily useful?

The most pressing question in today's world is: who is the supreme commander of your being? You might ask yourself whether it is you or your mind. To gain more control over our lives, we must be in a flow state to control our minds. These exercises will enable you to lift yourself, and you will be able to gain deep focus with these exercises.

Essentially, I want to convey here the mind is like technology. We can and should master the use of mind technology through various available techniques, which will be described in this book.

Brains can be compared to computer hardware in some ways. Just as computer hardware uses software to function effectively, the brain uses 20 like an operating system called the mind.

The most pressing question in today's world is: who is the supreme commander of your being? You might ask yourself whether it is you or your mind.

Super easy esercises......

Super
easy
exercises can
make anyone
at
any age more
intelligent

DNA

"

Can we use our
minds and our minds
as we want?

DNA   "

You can install super-fast software in your mind, you can do so with the help of the exercises provided.

The goal is to achieve a state of flow. Through my research, I have discovered a range of exercises that can help you get into a state of flow and focus. This set of activities will work in the brain in the same way as a software application. As a result, they will benefit you by increasing your attention speed, focusing, and avoiding distractions through different techniques.

Speaking metaphorically, connecting the dots will become more rapid,

This will allow you to perform better in the future. Let me tell you one important fact: the mind cannot be managed or mastered with simple thinking techniques most people use. In my experience, these exercises improve the mind's ability to focus and the speed at which the mind can pay prolonged attention.

Alternatively, one could say that just like the processors of computers have the potential to become faster and to perform more effectively and efficiently. Similarly, these exercise-driven flow states will increase the brain's capacity to process information manifolds at a super-fast pace.

Speaking metaphorically, connecting the dots will become more rapid, meaning that thinking will become faster. As we are in flow, we create original ideas by combining these facts quickly at high speeds to create novel ideas. This process enables the emergence of new concepts. A variety of techniques and exercises can be used to accomplish this.

It would be a fair description of the corpus callosum if one were to refer to it as a major brain bridge. It is like a big cable connecting two parts of the brain. In a way, it is similar to an internet cable. It is a bundle of over 200 million nerve fibres connecting the left and right lobes. Through this connection, communication can be

"

What is the
scientific secret to
self-talk?

"

DNA

established between the brain's two hemispheres. Like an internet cable, the speed of the brain's cables can be improved through multiple exercises.

Using both hands to write is recommended

I want to suggest an exercise that I think is unique and soulful, and I will explain why. Please write with both hands simultaneously. The activity is quite interesting. Initially, this will be challenging, but you can start with a single letter. For example, I suggest that you write the letter A with two hands simultaneously on two separate pages. Next, write the letter B, then write the letter C, then write the letter D, and so on. While learning this exciting exercise, you should write one alphabet at a time and move on to words as you progress. You can do it in your mind imagining it.

Leonardo Davinci, the master artist and painter of the Mona Lisa, used to do this. Undoubtedly, he was a genius and probably used various mental exercises to achieve that status. Hold a pen or pencil in your non-dominant hand as you would with your dominant hand and write with it as if it were your dominant hand. It would help if you used a hand other than your preferred one to operate the mouse on your computer. As a result of switching your mouse hand, your non-dominant hand will be more dexterous, increasing your productivity.

You can perform small daily tasks with your non-dominant hand without using your dominant hand. In addition to brushing your teeth with your non-dominant hand, you can open doors and put on accessories. Use your non-dominant hand as often as possible to make it more comfortable.

You can perform ......

You can perform
small daily
tasks with your
non-dominant
hand without
using your
dominant hand.

DNA

Imagining and visualizing- upside down

Imagining and visualizing- upside down, Da Vinci's upside-down method is another way of looking at things. In this very second one thing that you are watching right now. If you are looking at an object, immediately move your eyes to the top right corner of the thing that you are looking at. Thus, it should be rotated slowly to the right clockwise, so it slowly turns to the right. There comes the point when it is flipped upside down. If you do this, your mind can think outside the box. The ability to conceive original ideas will be at your disposal.

The eye was considered the most crucial organ in the body by Leonardo da Vinci. In his description, he says: "This is the eye, the one who leads all others". In my opinion, it is possible to trigger many neural circuits that can help us think outside the box if we use different ways of visualizing things a little differently from the typical routine ways of visualizing.

No image can enter the eye without being turned upside down," Leonardo discovered. However, he didn't know that the optic nerve transmits the image to the brain, flipping it right side up. Future scientists will solve this question.

Think out Loud and record your thoughts

This exercise can increase our thinking speed, brain power, and creativity. You can practice the habit of thinking aloud. Think and talk about a pre-selected topic of choice and interest, record those thoughts and listen back when possible. Discovering that your words start coming out of your mouth without thinking would be astounding. New comments in the form of ideas will start running ahead of your conscious thought. Talking out loud or self-talking

Da Vinci's upside-down......

Da Vinci's
upside-down
method is
another way of
looking at
things. In this
very second one
thing that you
are watching
right now.

DNA

is generally regarded as a social faux pas. Despite this, a recent study from Bangor University found that thinking aloud can have several positive effects. In addition, talking to yourself is considered a sign of intelligence.

We frequently speak silently to ourselves throughout the day, asking ourselves silent questions throughout the day, and it is not uncommon for us to do so. We must think aloud when managing our thoughts and emotions to gain better control over our introspection. When it comes to improving our reflection, this is crucial.

Brainstorming

is a process that involves generating ideas. To solve a problem or accomplish a task, an idea generator or brainstormer generates many ideas to solve the problem. It is possible to use several techniques when brainstorming ideas. There are several techniques you can use to help you brainstorm some ideas.

I believe that an essential part of this process is to come up with as many ideas as possible. Brainstorming is switching off your analytical left brain and turning on your intuitive right brain to generate original creative ideas. This is to come up with innovative solutions to problems. This refers to the point at which you put the pen on the paper and run it until it becomes tired. This is when whatever is in your head is transferred to paper.

You may ask yourself some of the following questions. Do I love what I do? Do I waste time without a purpose? Work/personal relationships: what's the right balance? Is there an opportunity that I am not pursuing that I should? In my life, what small thing will have the most significant impact? What is the most likely event in my life over the next six months?

We must think......

We must think
aloud when
managing our
thoughts and
emotions to gain
better control
over our
introspection.
When it comes to
improving our
reflection, this
is crucial.

DNA

Write with a free flow

White paper without lines works like magic. If you want to express yourself free-flowingly, you need to put pen to paper and let it run over the page for a long time without fearing your inner criticism. For writing to be successful, in generating ideas we need to focus on the topic, what we are thinking, and what we are writing instead of worrying about whether thoughts are related or not.

Let's get into the habit of writing more often. In the first stage, we should write for five minutes at a time. By doing this exercise, you can remove the wall between yourself, your mind, and your thoughts. There is something essential that I would like to share with you. The concept of neuroscience can be summed up in this way. We have a sophisticated scanner at the front of our brains that can block many of our thoughts. Unfortunately, this scanner often prevents us from processing many of our ideas.

The frontal lobe also stops us from having innovative ideas without noticing them. Having become accustomed to free-flowing writing, we can allow our thoughts to flow through our mind to our fingers and then from tip of the pen onto the magical white paper by writing in this manner. Using this exercise, we can also enter a state of mind that allows us to be most productive.

I have seen the personal diaries of some of the most creative scientists on the web. My research has revealed that most of these geniuses kept journals made of plain white paper with no lines in a landscape format. It will be possible for you to see what Einstein's diary looked like when it was written. Additionally, we can see what Leonardo's diary looked like during his lifetime. You can find pictures of their journals on search engines. You will be surprised to find out that they did not have any lines in their diaries, which surprised me.

You are imperceptibly and involuntarily prevented from writing, expressing, and representing your thoughts in their natural flow by lines. Therefore, writing in a diary without lines can be a unique and rewarding experience.

I have seen the......

I have seen the
personal diaries of
some of the most
creative scientists
on the web. My
research has
revealed that most
of these geniuses
kept journals made
of plain white
paper with no
lines in a
landscape format

DNA

Your life is filled with how many words? Research in this field may be conducted in the future. It is no secret that we usually use a maximum of a few hundred words when we think or speak. To my mind, every word we say, every word we think, and every word we write is loaded with a certain amount of energy. In addition, there is a sense of movement associated with it and a sense of energy. In the past, we were unaware that we could get so much energy from our words and thoughts. We couldn't generate this much power by any other means than through our words and ideas.

Humans cannot survive without words, just as they cannot survive without food or air. Good words are no less crucial for meaningful living than any other necessity. Air is essential for life as much as food is, and solid and articulate words are needed to ensure life's success. As a result of free-flow writing, we can make them more powerful.

Do Mirror writing!

Essentially, mirror-writing produces letters, words, or sentences in reverse order to appear normal when viewed in a mirror. Mirror writing may not be intentional for some people, but some children unintentionally do it.

Now, write it as if you were looking in the mirror. You can do that too. Try to image a word so that its reflection is being formed in the mirror, and you copy it in your mind's eye, for example, any letter such as the letter B or F. See it in your imagination and then draw it in your imagination. Or you can write it down.

The famous artist and painter Leonardo da Vinci wrote not only in a method of shorthand that he had invented but also in a method of writing in mirror image, beginning on the left and moving to the right. As a rule, he would only consistently write in the expected direction when writing something intended for someone else. Many people are unaware of the purpose of his mirror writing, but my neuroscientific intuitions suggest he uses it to enhance his flow state.

The famous artist and painter......

The famous
artist and
painter
Leonardo da Vinci
wrote not only
in a method of
shorthand that he
had invented but
also in a
method of writing in
mirror image,
beginning on the
left and
moving to the right.

DNA

bc1abbdc-6737-4995-be6e-aa677e7a7cc6R01